101 AMAZING USES for

COCONUT OiL

FAMILIUS

FOR SADIE AND MATTHEW

Published by Familius LLC, www.familius.com

Familius books are available at special discounts for bulk purchases, whether for sales promotions or for family or corporate use. For more information, contact Familius Sales at 559-876-2170 or email orders@familius.com.

DISCLAIMER: The material in this book is for informational purposes only. It is not intended to be a substitute for professional medical advice, diagnosis, or treatment. Always seek the advice of your physician or other qualified healthcare provider with any questions you may have regarding a medical condition or treatment. Never disregard professional medical advice or delay in seeking it because of something you have read in this book.

Library of Congress Cataloging-in-Publication Data
2017933384

Print ISBN 9781945547140
Ebook ISBN 9781945547577

Printed in the United States of America

Edited by Lindsay Sandberg
Cover design by David Miles
Book design by Brooke Jorden and David Miles

10 9 8 7 6 5 4 3 2 1
First Edition

101 AMAZING USES for COCONUT OIL

DECREASE WRINKLES, BALANCE HORMONES, CLEAN A HAIRBRUSH, AND 98 MORE!

Susan Branson

CONTENTS

INTRODUCTION

IT'S ROUND; IT'S HAIRY; IT'S A COCONUT!

Coconuts are the fruit of the coconut palm tree that measure anywhere from five to ten inches across. The outer husk is made up of tough fibers and has a hairy appearance. When young, the husk is green, but it turns gray or brown as it matures. The white coconut meat inside the husk is used to make coconut oil. There are two distinct types of coconuts. One has an elongated shape so it can dig into sand, a very fibrous husk to protect the seed, and only a small amount of water to make it buoyant for ocean dispersal. Over time, human cultivation of coconuts led to the second type, which we commonly find in grocery stores today. They are round with more water and a greater meat-to-husk ratio.

Indonesia is the largest producer of coconuts today, followed by the Philippines and India. In these cultures, and many others, coconuts form a staple in the diet. The entire fruit is highly nutritious, and the coconut oil, meat, milk, and water are used for their vitamin, mineral, fiber, and fat content. Coconut oil contains polyphenols, which give the oil its unique fragrance and sweet taste. Polyphenols are also antimicrobial and potent antioxidants. They protect the body from pathogens and prevent reactive oxygen compounds from causing extensive damage in the body.

Coconut oil is one of the most concentrated sources of energy and contains 120 calories per tablespoon. The oil is the primary source of fat in the fruit and is responsible for most of its calories. It is composed mainly of medium-chain fatty acids like lauric acid, capric acid, caprylic acid, palmitic acid, and myristic acid. These are antimicrobial and are powerful compounds that help stave off infection and disease. Medium-chain fatty acids don't act like other fatty acids. The majority of fats and oils we consume are long-chain fatty acids, like those found in meat, milk, eggs, and most vegetable oils. They are implicated in heart disease and obesity. The medium-chain fatty acids found in coconut oil do not have the same effects. In fact, they are cardioprotective and are not implicated in weight gain. These fatty acids are absorbed directly from the intestine into the blood where they are transported to the liver and used for energy. Long-chain fatty acids, on the other hand, are stored in fat tissue if they are not used immediately. No wonder coconut oil is known as the healthiest of the fats and oils!

WHERE DID YOU COME FROM, COCONUT?

Coconut palms are found on every tropical coast and are synonymous with dream vacations promising beaches, sun, and relaxation. Despite the ubiquitous nature of coconut palm trees today, they actually originated from two distinct populations of coconuts long ago. The first was in Southeast Asia (Pacific coconuts), and the other was on the outer edge of Southern India (Indian Ocean coconuts). Ancient Austronesians introduced Pacific coconuts to Madagascar and east Africa thousands of years ago while traveling along their trade routes, giving rise to a genetically mixed coconut in that region. It wasn't until much later in time that coconuts found their way into Europe by way of Portuguese sailors. They discovered coconuts during their seafaring travels and brought them to the west coast of Africa where they flourished in plantations. Later, travelers carried them aboard their ships to Brazil and the Caribbean. Coconuts on the west side of the New World tropics were from Southeast Asia, brought by Austronesians traveling west rather than east.

Every tropical region has a special story of their coconut origins. Many are buried deep within history, but there is one that depicts how coconuts made their way to Florida. A ship named Providencia was on its way from Trinidad to Spain. On board were 20,000 coconuts. On January 9, 1878, the sailors were enjoying a little too much drink and were not as attentive to their voyage as they should have been. The ship ran aground off the coast of what is now Palm Beach. By way of apology, they gave the locals their cargo of coconuts. The coconuts were planted in their new location, and palm trees sprouted. The area was aptly named Palm Beach. Today, this fruit is now grown in more than seventy countries around the world and is used for food, shelter, tools, and fuel.

The Portuguese gave the coconuts their name. When sailors first saw coconuts, they thought they looked like heads because of their round shape and three holes, giving the appearance of eyes and a mouth. They called the fruit "coco," which has since been adopted by Western European languages and is known as "coconut" in English. Others believe the sailors used the name "Coco" because the coconut looked like the head of a ghostly folklore figure that kidnapped children. Parents used the threat of "Coco" to scare children into being obedient. The coconut also has a prominent place in Indian rituals. They are a symbol of prosperity and are put on both sides of entrances to temples, homes, and workplaces. Fishermen offer coconuts to the seas, hoping to catch an abundance of fish.

Asian and Pacific cultures value the coconut palm so highly that they call it the "Tree of Life." They believe it has special healing properties and use it as a medicine in a wide variety of illness. They are not alone. Cultures all over the world have been using coconuts to restore vitality. Today, the use of coconut is being extensively studied to determine whether long-held beliefs in coconut's therapeutic value is warranted. Turns out, it is.

....

YOu BoUGHT IT. NOW WHAT?

The last two decades saw a rise in popularity of edible coconut oil and an increase in availability in stores and online. For years, all saturated fats were labeled as unhealthy, but we now know that the type of saturated fat in coconut oil has many therapeutic benefits when used in moderation.

When shopping for coconut oil, there are several different kinds to choose from, depending on how they are processed. Generally speaking, there are refined and virgin coconut oils. Refined oils are produced from copra, coconut removed from the shell and dried into an inedible form that is smoky and dirty. They are further refined by bleaching and steam deodorizing to produce coconut oils that have very little flavor and taste. This process keeps all the medium-chain fatty acids intact but tends to result in oil lower in antioxidants than virgin coconut oils. Refined coconut oils still possess many of the medicinal properties of virgin oils—with the exception of liquid coconut oil. Coconut oil remains solidified up to 76 degrees Fahrenheit, turning into a liquid at temperatures higher than this. Liquid coconut oil remains a liquid even at low temperatures due to the removal of lauric acid. This is the major fatty acid in coconut and is responsible for most of its therapeutic benefits. Don't purchase this oil if its intended use is to improve health. Hydrogenated coconut oil is another refined coconut oil to avoid for consumption. The unsaturated fats in this oil are con-verted into trans fats, so the oil will remain solid above 76 degrees

Fahrenheit. Trans fats are indisputably poor dietary fats and are implicated in heart disease.

Virgin coconut oils begin with fresh coconut, not the dried copra of refined coconut oils. When choosing virgin oil, make sure copra is not the starting point. There is no certification body monitoring the labeling of coconut oils, so any company can call their coconut oil "virgin." There is also no difference between the labels "extra virgin" and "virgin" coconut oil. Virgin coconut oils are produced from pressing the oil out of dried or wet fresh coconut meat, and both have higher antioxidant levels than refined coconut oils[1] and the characteristic coconut smell and taste. They are not bleached, deodorized, or refined. It is interesting to note that coconut oils labeled as "raw" or "cold-pressed" have less antioxidants than ones extracted by heat. [2] Organic products are always advisable to reduce the toxic load, but pesticide levels in coconuts have not been detected.[3] One concern, however, is the emergence of GMO coconuts. The chemical makeup of these coconuts is different and may decrease the therapeutic value or affect the body in adverse ways.

Coconut oil can be kept in the cupboard at room temperature where it will remain fresh for about six months. It can be used in cooking, baking, coating nonstick pans, and adding flavor to food. For health purposes, it can be consumed directly or added to hot beverages. As a cosmetic, the oil can be applied to the skin, hair, nails, mouth, eyes, or any other place deemed necessary. When applying to the body, ensure the coconut oil is not contaminated with other ingredients. Always use a clean spoon when dipping into the jar.

Coconut oil can readily be made at home. Open a coconut purchased from your local market. Pour the coconut milk into a jar and save for another use. Scrape out the coconut meat and place in a blender. Add two times the amount of water over the coconut meat. Blend on medium-low for a minute, then switch the setting to high until a smooth, creamy consistency has been reached. Pour this liquid through several layers of cheesecloth into a bowl. Squeeze the liquid from the cheesecloth and throw it away. Cover the bowl and put it in a dark place for several days. Next, put the bowl in a warm, lighted area and allow the oil to separate from the liquid. Once separation is complete, put the bowl in the refrigerator. The coconut oil will solidify and can be scooped out and stored in a jar.

IS COCONUT OIL SAFE?

Consuming coconut oil is regarded as safe in amounts normally found in the diet. Studies using amounts up to 2 tablespoons a day for adults and 2 teaspoons a day for children have been well tolerated. Allergic reactions can happen but appear significantly less often than with other food items.[4] When psyllium—a dietary fiber—is consumed with coconut oil, the absorption of the fatty acids is reduced. Coconut oil should not be taken alongside psyllium if the oil is intended for therapeutic use. No interactions with other herbs, supplements, drugs, or foods are known.[5]

TIPS TO GET ALL THE BENEFITS, DAILY.

It takes commitment to consume 2 or 3 tablespoons of coconut oil each and every day. The easiest way is to eat it right off the spoon. Coconut oil has a light, creamy texture that melts quickly for easy swallowing. Some people don't like to eat the oil neat, so here are ten other ways to incorporate it into the daily diet.

1. Mix it into warm breakfast cereals like oatmeal, grits, and creamed wheat.
2. Replace the oil that has separated and is sitting on top of natural peanut butter with an equivalent amount of coconut oil. Mix thoroughly.
3. Drizzle it over popcorn.
4. Mix it into warm rice, pasta, or mashed potatoes.
5. Use it as an ingredient in homemade ice cream.
6. Substitute 1 tablespoon coconut oil for an egg in baking recipes.
7. Replace canola oil with an equal amount of coconut oil in homemade mayonnaise.
8. Sip a drink of 1 tablespoon coconut oil, the juice of half a lemon, and warm water.
9. Top toast, muffins, biscuits, and crackers.
10. Substitute for butter in brownies, cookies, cakes, and loaves.

CHAPTER 1

MORNING WAKE-UP TO EVENING INDULGENCE

NUTRITION

HEALTH

WELL-BEING

BEAUTY

1. COFFEE

The aroma of coffee wafting through the house is just the incentive many need to throw off the covers and slide out of bed. The caffeine in coffee stimulates the brain by increasing energy metabolism and enhancing mood. Many people add milk, cream, or sugar to their coffee. Dairy promotes mucus formation, and sugar can depress the immune system. Avoid these pitfalls while still getting a great cup of coffee by substituting coconut oil. Add 1 or 2 teaspoons into freshly brewed coffee and stir until it has melted. Pour into a blender and turn to high for five seconds. This step is important to really mix the coconut oil into the coffee. Simply stirring can leave little dots of oil on the surface of the coffee that are not very appealing.

Coconut oil improves the metabolism of fats and reduces their storage in fat tissue.[6] It encourages overall weight reduction, particularly in the abdominal area, and increases energy.[7] Coconut oil even nourishes the brain to enhance concentration and focus. The medium-chain fatty acids in the oil cross the blood-brain barrier where they are oxidized and used as a fuel source.[8] Adding coconut oil to coffee will lift the mind's morning fog and rev up the body's metabolism to provide mental clarity and physical energy.

2. COOKING AT HIGH HEAT

The high saturated fat content of coconut oil makes it ideal to use in cooking over the stovetop. It has a high smoke point, or the temperature at which the oil begins to give off a continuous wisp of smoke. The higher the smoke point, the more suited the oil is to cooking with heat. As oil heats, it is susceptible to oxidation, producing an off flavor in the oil and in the food being cooked. More importantly, however, when oil oxidizes, it produces compounds that may be toxic to the body, causing inflammation and damage. The more saturated the fat or oil is, the higher it can be heated before producing these offensive products. Coconut oil is more than 90 percent saturated, so using it to shallow-fry or sauté will ensure the intended flavors are reached without a detriment to health. Try this side dish using coconut oil to bring the ingredients together.

CRUNCHY LEMON QUINOA AND ASPARAGUS BOWL
ALLRECIPES.COM

1 pound fresh asparagus, trimmed
2 teaspoons coconut oil
1/2 onion, diced
2 cloves garlic, minced
1 cup cooked red quinoa
1/2 cup low-sodium vegetable stock
1 tablespoon ground turmeric
1/2 cup nutritional yeast
Juice of 1/2 large lemon

1. Fill a saucepan halfway with water; bring to a boil. Add aspara-
    gus and cook uncovered until tender but still crispy, about 2–3
    minutes. Drain in a colander and rinse with cold water to stop
    the cooking process.
2. Heat coconut oil in a large skillet over medium heat. Add
    the onion and garlic; cook until onion is translucent, about
    5 minutes. Stir in cooked quinoa, vegetable stock, and tur-
    meric. Cook until flavors combine, about 5–6 minutes. Stir in
    blanched asparagus, nutritional yeast, and lemon juice. Cook
    and stir for 3–4 minutes.

3. DIETARY FAT

Fats are nutrients essential to perform an abundance of functions
in the body. They enhance the bioavailability of fat-soluble micro-
nutrients and make up structural components in cell membranes
and around nerves. Fats form hormones to regulate the body's activities and are a concentrated source of energy. They provide a
protective cushion around organs and insulation under the skin.
Without an adequate supply of fats, the body could not function
properly.

The overwhelming majority of fats consumed consists of long-
chain fatty acids and are found in meat, fish, dairy, nuts, and seeds.
Included in this category are commonly used oils like olive, canola, safflower, and peanut. These fats are digested and made into
triglycerides before entering the bloodstream. They are carried to
fat cells for storage until they are needed for fuel. Many of these
long-chain fatty acids are known to increase heart disease by

elevating low-density lipoprotein cholesterol (LDL), known as bad cholesterol.[9] Coconut oil, on the other hand, is made up mostly of medium-chain fatty acids. These acids are directly absorbed from the small intestine into the bloodstream without being digested. They go to the liver and can be used immediately by the body for energy instead of being shunted into fat cells for storage. When consumed in moderation, medium-chain fatty acids actually help increase metabolism,[10] decrease body weight,[11] and raise the body's high-density lipoprotein cholesterol (HDL)—also known as the good cholesterol.[12] Substituting coconut oil for other fats and oils in the diet can protect the cardiovascular system and aid in weight loss.

4. EGG FRESHNESS

Eggs are eaten for breakfast, lunch, and dinner. They are used in both sweet and savory dishes, whether as the star of the show or as a welcome side dish. Eggs provide a low-calorie meal that is high in nutrients and flavor. Consequently, eggs are a staple in many homes and find their way onto almost every shopping list. The USDA recommends consuming eggs within five weeks after laying. Typically, eggs take a few days to reach the supermarket shelves and can sit there for weeks before being purchased. Over time, the freshness of eggs decreases, which can impact flavor. If left long enough, bacteria can break down the protein and create hydrogen sulfide gas, commonly known as the rotten egg smell.

To preserve freshness, cover the eggs in a small amount of coconut oil. Eggs have thousands of tiny pores in the shell that can

NUTRITION

let in oxygen or bacteria. By sealing the pores with coconut oil, the egg is protected inside the shell and freshness is extended for several weeks.

5. HOMEMADE CHOCOLATE

Chocolate inspires feelings of happiness and well-being in those who have conditioned their body to release dopamine as a reward for indulging in this sweet confection. This makes it very difficult to pass an aisle of chocolate bars or a pan of brownies on the counter without satisfying the craving a little. Every time we eat chocolate, we reinforce the positive feedback loop that releases dopamine in the brain and makes us feel good. This is a good thing, as long as chocolate is eaten in moderation. Too much can cause weight gain, but more distressing are the unhealthy compounds ingested with the average chocolate bar. Corn syrup and sugar are often the main ingredients. Hydrogenated oils, preservatives, and natural and artificial flavors usually make the list, too. These depress the immune system, are bad for the heart, and increase the workload of the liver. You may think natural flavors are okay, but often, they're not. They begin with an ingredient found in nature, but by the time they are added to the food, they have been refined and altered to the point where they little resemble the starting product.

Chocolate cravings can be satisfied while still getting a dopamine boost and consuming ingredients that nourish the body.

HEALTH

WELL-BEING

BEAUTY

HOMEMADE MELT-IN-YOUR-MOUTH DARK CHOCOLATE (PALEO)
ALLRECIPES.COM

1/2 cup coconut oil
1/2 cup cocoa powder
3 tablespoons honey
1/2 teaspoon vanilla extract

1. Gently melt coconut oil in a saucepan over medium-low heat. Stir cocoa powder, honey, and vanilla extract into melted oil until well blended.
2. Pour mixture into a candy mold or pliable tray.
3. Refrigerate until chilled, about 1 hour. Keep any leftovers in the refrigerator to maintain their shape.

NUTRITION

HEALTH

WELL-BEING

BEAUTY

CHAPTER 2

MANAGING DISEASE

NUTRITION

HEALTH

WELL-BEING

BEAUTY

6. ALZHEIMER'S

Alzheimer's disease—a form of dementia—is a progressive brain disorder that is irreversible. It can begin with greater memory loss and result in wandering and getting lost, repeating questions, and some personality and behavioral changes. As it progresses, memory loss and confusion grow worse and people may have trouble recognizing friends and family, carrying out multistep tasks, or coping with new situations. In the late stage, brain tissue shrinks significantly and communication becomes difficult. Alzheimer's patients become completely dependent on others for care and often become bedridden. In most people with Alzheimer's, symptoms begin in their midsixties. Early onset may have genetic factors in play, and late onset arises from complex brain changes that occur over decades. Current treatment approaches encourage patients to focus on mental function and manage behavioral symptoms. Several medications have been approved by the United States FDA for the treatment of these symptoms.

Coconut oil has been shown to increase the survival of brain nerve cells treated with amyloid-β (Aβ) peptide. Aβ peptide consists of the amino acids that make up a plaque in the brains of Alzheimer's patients that cause nerve cell death and the degeneration of brain function.[13] Coconut oil can also work indirectly to slow the progression of Alzheimer's. The medium-chain fatty acids in coconut oil are converted into ketones by the liver. Ketones can be used by the brain as an alternate source of energy. This is important because the ability of the brain in Alzheimer's patients to supply glucose for energy declines and, along with it, brain function. Having an alternate source of energy can keep the brain's metabolic functions moving forward. Coconut oil can provide the medium-chain fatty acids necessary to increase the amount of ketones in the blood. Oral administration of ketones showed elevated levels in the blood in mild to moderate Alzheimer's patients and significant improvements in cognitive scores.[14] These results were confirmed by another study that demonstrated improvements in mood, self-care, daily activity performance, and cognition after patients were administered a ketogenic agent for a prolonged period.[15] Consuming coconut oil on its own each day or as an ingredient in meals can provide the brain with fuel for energy-starved nerve cells and slow the progression of Alzheimer's disease.

7. ARTHRITIS

Arthritis is the most common disability in the United States,[16] affecting more than fifty million people. There are many types, but the two most common are osteoarthritis and rheumatoid arthritis.

Osteoarthritis is characterized by inflammation of the joints. The joints provide the connection between bones that allow for movement. They are cushioned by cartilage to allow the joint to move smoothly and easily. In osteoarthritis, the cartilage breaks down and causes inflammation. Extra fluid is produced in the joint, resulting in swelling. This disease affects many people as they age due to natural wear and tear. Heredity plays a role, as does injury from trauma or disease. Those afflicted suffer from joints that are painful, creaky, stiff, and swollen. Their range of motion is reduced, particularly in the hands, feet, spine, hips, and knees. Reducing the stress on the joint cartilage is recommended to alleviate some of the symptoms. This involves losing weight and avoiding certain activities. The goal of treatment is to reduce pain and inflammation to allow for more comfortable movement. Medications are taken as pills, creams, gels, and even injections into the arthritic joint. Side effects of these can include gastrointestinal distress such as stomach upset, diarrhea, or ulcers.

Rheumatoid arthritis is an autoimmune disorder in which the immune system mistakenly attacks its own body tissues. The lining of the joints become painfully swollen and can lead to bone erosion and joint deformity over time. Symptoms can spread to other non-joint tissues of the body. It's not known what causes this disease, but genetics combined with environmental triggers are suspected. This chronic disease is without a cure and is managed mostly through medications. Nonsteroidal anti-inflammatory drugs, steroids, or disease-modifying antirheumatic drugs can be prescribed to reduce pain, swelling, and joint damage. Possible side effects include digestive problems, liver and kidney damage, heart problems, thinning of bones, diabetes, weight gain, and severe lung infections.

Virgin coconut oil contains polyphenols that are known antioxidants. These chemicals can stop the action of reactive oxygen species and free radicals that cause joint degradation in both osteoarthritis and rheumatoid arthritis.[17] When polyphenols from virgin coconut oil were used to treat arthritic rats, swelling was greatly reduced after three weeks of treatment. Antioxidant levels were increased, and markers of inflammation were decreased.[18] It is important to consume virgin coconut oil to help alleviate the symptoms of arthritis because this type has intact polyphenols.

Refined coconut oil would not be as effective, as most of the poly-phenols have been removed.[19] It still has the medium-chain fatty acids intact, however, and these, too, are anti-inflammatory com-pounds that can aid in reducing swelling associated with arthritis.

8. BEAVER FEVER

Giardia is a microscopic parasite found in soil, food, or water that has been contaminated with feces from infected animals or humans. This parasite is found worldwide, often in areas of poor sanitation, and is a common cause of waterborne illness—called "beaver fever"—in the United States. It lurks in lakes and streams, but it can also be found in municipal water, hot tubs, and swim-ming pools. Once ingested, *Giardia* parasites live in the intestines and cause intestinal illness, resulting in cramps, bloating, nausea, and diarrhea. Infection can last for several weeks, but it is not uncommon for intestinal problems to continue for longer. Not ev-eryone experiences symptoms, so some may pass on the parasite unknowingly. If the symptoms are severe, antibiotics can be taken to eliminate the parasite. Nausea and a metallic taste in the mouth are common side effects to the antibiotics.

When *Giardia* affects humans, it can cause nutritional deficien-cies in children, weight loss, and an impaired immune system. Because it can last so long and have lingering effects, eliminating the infection early is greatly desired. Lauric acid from coconut oil has been found to be effective in treating beaver fever in hamsters. Infected hamsters were divided into groups and given equal doses of either a common antibiotic used to treat beaver fever, lauric acid from coconut oil, or a combination of both. Lauric acid on its own was able to eliminate up to 82 percent of the parasites. Combined with the antibiotic, lauric acid eliminated up to 98 percent.[20] This was more effective than the antibiotic alone. Using lauric acid along with the antibiotic would cut the antibiotic dose in half, which benefits the good intestinal bacteria and reduces the risk of side effects.

9. BREAST CANCER

Breast cancer starts when cells of the breast begin to grow out of control and form a tumor. Tumors are cancerous if they grow and spread into other areas of the body. It is much more common in women, but men can get breast cancer too. Early detection can be made through mammograms before symptoms begin. If not detected early, breast cancer can cause bloody discharge from the nipple or changes in the shape or texture of the breast or nipple. It can also be felt as a lump. Treatment may involve radiation, chemotherapy, or surgery.

Chemotherapy can disrupt the lives of patients and reduce their quality of life. This is a very difficult time, and any improvement in the side effects of treatment and on the outlook of life can impact overall wellness. Coconut oil was given to stage III and IV breast cancer patients undergoing chemotherapy to determine any effect it may have on patients' quality of life. A second group was used as a control and not given coconut oil. Those patients consuming coconut oil reported having more energy, better sleep, improved appetite, and less breathing difficulties compared to the control group. Body image, breast symptoms, and future perspectives were also improved in the test group. Symptoms related to the side effects of chemotherapy were reduced with the consumption of coconut oil.[21]

Coconut oil also shows promise as an anticancer agent in breast cancer cells. Two of the fatty acids found in coconut oil—capric and caproic acids—were used to treat cancerous breast cells for forty-eight hours. They were able to reduce the viability of the cancerous cells by up to 80 percent compared to cancer cells not treated with the fatty acids.[22]

10. BRONCHITIS

Bronchitis is a respiratory disease characterized by the inflammation of the lining of the bronchial airways of the lungs. Acute bronchitis is a viral infection that can result from a cold or other respiratory infection and causes the mucous membranes to swell and air pathways to narrow. Chronic bronchitis is more severe and is a constant inflammation of the lining of the bronchial tubes, most often caused by smoking. People with bronchitis have coughing spells and often cough up mucus. Chest pain, fever, chills, and fatigue are other symptoms. Acute bronchitis often goes away on its own after a short time, while chronic bronchitis persists and often requires antibiotics, cough medicine, or asthma inhalers.

When bronchitis is viral is origin, coconut oil can be used to assist the body in fighting the infection. The most abundant fatty acid in coconut oil is lauric acid. When this is ingested, it gets converted to monolaurin in the body. Monolaurin attacks enveloped viruses such as the bronchitis virus. The envelope of a bronchitis

NUTRITION

HEALTH

WELL-BEING

BEAUTY

virus is a protective covering that fuses with a host cell membrane and allows the virus to inject its genetic material into the host. The host cell is now infected, and the virus replicates itself many times before destroying its host. The viruses are released, and the infection spreads. Monolaurin dissolves the envelope of the virus and interrupts the signal that allows the host cell to be receptive to binding with the virus.[23] The virus is then unable to inject its genetic material into the host cell for replication, effectively preventing the virus from spreading. Consuming a few teaspoons of coconut oil each day, in smoothies, on toast with sea salt, or even straight out of the jar should boost the body's ability to fight bronchial viruses by having molecules ready to attenuate the spread of infection. Symptoms should clear more quickly, reducing inflammation and easing cough and congestion.

11. CAMPYLOBACTERIOSIS

Campylobacteriosis is an infectious disease caused by *Campylobacter* bacteria and is one of the most common causes of diarrhea worldwide. It is spread to humans most often through consuming undercooked poultry or from cross-contamination with other food. It's very important to clean cutting boards, utensils, cloths, and other surfaces that raw chicken comes into contact with to minimize the risk of infection. It doesn't take much to get sick. Even as few as five hundred *Campylobacter* organisms can infect a person. That's just one drop of raw chicken juice! A few years ago, a sampling of raw chicken from grocery stores found that 47 percent of the chicken was contaminated with *Campylobacter* organisms.[24] If ingested, these bacteria can produce bloody diarrhea, fever, and stomach cramps. Symptoms usually begin two to five days after infection and typically last about a week. Drinking plenty of fluids and getting rest should help recovery. Antibiotics are given only in severe cases or to people with weakened immune systems.

The most common species of *Campylobacter* that infects humans is *C. jejuni*. If contracted, the symptoms can bring misery, but the duration of the illness can be shortened by consuming coconut oil. Once in the body, capric acid from coconut oil is converted into monocaprin. Monocaprin is extremely effective at destroying *Campylobacter* and was found to reduce viable bacterial counts by 99.9 percent in one minute at room temperature. Not only that, but monocaprin has broad anticampylobacter activity and is effective against several different strains.[25] If food poisoning is suspected, take 1 teaspoon of coconut oil several times a day. If the symptoms are more severe, take up to 3 tablespoons a day in divided doses.

12. CHLAMYDIA

Chlamydia is a common sexually transmitted bacterial disease with over 1.5 million reported cased in the United States in 2015.[26] The actual number is much higher because many cases go undetected and unreported. Many people do not experience any symptoms and don't know they have it. Actually, only 10 percent of men and 30 percent of women develop symptoms.[27, 28] When they do appear, women report vaginal discharge, bleeding, frequent urination, and abdominal or pelvic pain. Men may experience painful urination, tender testicles, or mucus penile discharge.

NUTRITION

HEALTH

WELL-BEING

BEAUTY

If this disease is left untreated, it can cause serious complications. Fallopian tubes and the uterus may become permanently damaged in women. Infected mothers can pass the bacteria to their babies during birth, and the infection can cause preterm delivery.[29] Both men and women may experience inflammation of the liver or reactive arthritis. Fortunately, chlamydia is easily treated with antibiotics. Unfortunately, any damage done cannot be repaired.

The danger with chlamydia lies in its asymptomatic nature and widespread occurrence. Many people contract this disease and don't know they have it. They may go for prolonged periods without treatment, which allows the virus to spread and infect multiple organs of the body, causing irreversible and serious damage. The risk of spreading the disease to multiple partners also increases over time. However, ingesting coconut oil on a regular basis or using it as a vaginal lubricant or genital moisturizer can expose chlamydia bacteria to coconut oil's potent antibacterial compounds. Of these, lauric acid, capric acid, and monocaprin (converted from capric acid in the body) were tested for their effect on chlamydia bacteria and were found to rapidly inactivate them, causing a significant reduction in numbers.[30] The fatty acids destroyed the bacteria by injuring their protective outer membranes. Bacteria were prevented from replicating, and death quickly followed. Coconut oil can be used as a preventative in sexually active individuals and may destroy chlamydia bacteria before infection takes hold.

13. COLON CANCER

Colon cancer begins with the formation of benign clumps of cells called polyps in the large intestine. Over time, these polyps can become cancerous. In the early stages, lack of symptoms is common, but as the disease progresses, patients experience changes in bowel habits, rectal bleeding, abdominal pain, fatigue, and unexplained weight loss. Like most cancers, treatment is often radiation, chemotherapy, surgery, or a combination of these.

It is difficult to avoid toxins in the environment, so it is wise to take steps to ensure the body has the necessary compounds it needs to prevent tumors from forming. One class of these protective compounds is antioxidants. The phenolic acids in coconut oil are known antioxidants. Consuming phenolic compounds increases antioxidant protection within the body and can reduce cancer risk and the formation of tumors.[31]

It's not only coconut oil's antioxidants that are stars but also its fatty acids, lauric acid and palmitic acid. These abundant compounds, accounting for almost 60 percent of the fatty acids in coconut oil, were found to be strong growth inhibitors of three lines of human colon cancer cells.[32] Coconut oil shows promise as an effective antitumor agent and chemotherapeutic agent. Consuming a tablespoon of coconut oil a day may help reduce the viability of colon cancer cells and can be used as a preventative measure or as part of a therapeutic protocol.

NUTRITION

HEALTH

WELL-BEING

BEAUTY

NUTRITION

HEALTH

WELL-BEING

BEAUTY

14. CROHN'S DISEASE

Crohn's disease is a chronic inflammatory bowel disease affecting sections of the lining of the digestive tract, particularly the deep tissue of the small bowel and beginning of the colon. Symptoms develop gradually and can flare up suddenly or disappear for periods of time. Many people with Crohn's suffer from stomach pain and cramps, diarrhea, poor appetite, rectal bleeding, fatigue, and fever. While some with Crohn's disease find it runs in their family, most discover no such genetic link. The cause is unknown, but viral or bacterial infections may trigger the immune system, setting off an abnormal response, causing the immune system to attack cells of the digestive tract. In severe cases, surgery is sometimes indicated for treatment, but most patients are treated with anti-inflammatory or immune-suppressing drugs to reduce inflammation or antibiotics to kill harmful intestinal bacteria. Some side effects of these treatments include nausea, diarrhea, heartburn, headache, high blood pressure, diabetes, glaucoma, cancers, and liver damage.

This disease can be very debilitating and severely impact the quality of life of those afflicted. Taking traditional medications does help, but some of the potential side effects are dangerous. Coconut oil is safe and nontoxic and can be consumed to reduce inflammation of the colon and alleviate many of the symptoms of Crohn's disease. A study in mice fed either sunflower oil or a mixture of sunflower and coconut oil found that the colons of mice in the latter group had less inflammation.[33] It is thought that the medium-chain fatty acids in coconut oil were responsible for the reduction in intestinal inflammation and that these compounds could have a therapeutic effect in human Crohn's disease.

In cases where foreign bacteria or viruses are responsible for triggering inflammation in the digestive tract, coconut oil's anti-microbial compounds may reduce inflammation by destroying the invaders. The immune response would ease, swelling would lessen, and intestinal tissues would be soothed. Diets replacing some of the long-chain fatty acids with medium-chain fatty acids, like those found in coconut oil, would be beneficial in reducing intestinal inflammation and associated symptoms.

15. DIABETES

Diabetes is a disease that affects the way the body handles glucose, resulting in high levels of this sugar in the blood. There is type 1 diabetes, in which the pancreas produces little or no insulin, type 2 diabetes, in which the pancreas does produce insulin but the body doesn't use it as well as it should, and gestational diabetes, a form of high blood sugar affecting pregnant women. Some people are genetically predisposed to diabetes, but being overweight is also a risk factor. Feelings of thirst, frequent urination, fatigue, tingling, numbness in the hands or feet, and blurry vision are all signs of diabetes. Managing diabetes involves exercising, improving diet, and monitoring blood glucose levels. For many, daily insulin injections are needed.

Diabetics have to monitor their blood sugar levels to ensure they are not too high. Virgin coconut oil was shown to significantly reduce fasting blood glucose levels in diabetic male rats when administered orally once a day for four weeks. Oral glucose tolerance was also improved as well as serum insulin in one of the coconut treatment arms.[34] This hypoglycemic and enhanced insulin secretion activity shows virgin coconut oil has promise as a therapeutic agent in the management of blood sugar in diabetic patients.

Diabetics also have to be careful of too little blood sugar as well. This is known as hypoglycemia and can result in confusion, trouble talking, and clumsiness, among other issues. It's important to get blood sugar up quickly by eating foods high in simple sugars. The problem is that sometimes the person doesn't realize they are hypoglycemic or it is so severe that they cannot correct it on their own and need help. It is not uncommon for diabetic patients to occasionally be hypoglycemic.

Consuming the medium-chain fatty acids found in coconut oil can dramatically lessen the cognitive decline that happens with hypoglycemia. Eleven diabetic patients with hypoglycemia were given either a medium-chain fatty acid drink or a placebo drink before undergoing a series of cognitive tests. The medium-chain fatty acid drink greatly improved brain function on all tests. These acids supported synaptic nerve transmissions in the brain under low glucose levels. Nerve function in diabetic hypoglycemic patients is normally disrupted under these conditions, leading to a decline in cognition.[35] The medium-chain fatty acids were likely converted to ketones in the body and transported to the glucose-starved brain where they were used as an alternate fuel source so the brain could continue to function optimally. Coconut oil can act as a preventative to preserve brain function during episodes of hypoglycemia in diabetic patients.

16. EPILEPSY

Epilepsy is a disorder of the central nervous system affecting nerve activity in the brain. Groups of nerves can send out the wrong signal and result in a seizure. Some seizures are small and can go unnoticed, while others involve violent muscle contractions and loss of consciousness. Altered emotions and perceptions are common and may cause strange behavior for brief periods. Genetics plays a role in some types of epilepsy, making the person more sensitive to particular triggers that can cause seizures. Brain damage or head injuries may also cause this condition, but in about half of epileptic patients, no known cause has been identified. Doctors generally treat epilepsy with medication to reduce the frequency and intensity of seizures. These come with a list of side effects from mild challenges, like fatigue, to severe problems, such as suicidal thoughts and behaviors. Surgery is warranted in some cases, but this, as always, comes with inherent risks.

Coconut oil contains a high percentage of medium-chain fatty acids. When coconut oil is ingested, the medium-chain fatty acids are absorbed into the blood where they go to the liver. The liver is then able to convert these into ketones. A recent study found that administering a ketogenic diet to epileptic children for three months significantly lowered the number of seizures compared to epileptic children who were not fed this diet. This was effective regardless of the type of epilepsy.[36] Consuming coconut oil provides the necessary compounds to form ketones in the body that can attenuate epileptic seizures and reduce the need for antiseizure medications.

NUTRITION

HEALTH

WELL-BEING

BEAUTY

17. E. COLI POISONING

Escherichia coli is a bacterium that normally lives in the intestines of humans and animals. Many types of *E. coli* are harmless and are important to the health of the digestive tract. Several species, however, are pathogenic and cause bloody diarrhea, urinary tract infections, anemia, or kidney failure. Contraction of *E. coli* can be made from contact with infected persons or animals or from consuming food or water containing the bacteria. *E. coli* can contaminate meat during processing, and if it is not cooked to 160 degrees Fahrenheit, it can survive and infect the consumer. Sometimes, cows spread the bacteria to their milk as it passes their udders. If the milk is not pasteurized, the bacteria will continue to live and pose a threat. Even raw fruits and vegetables can have *E. coli* bacteria from contact with contaminated water or persons. Three or four days after ingesting *E. coli*, food poisoning becomes evident as symptoms develop. They usually subside on their own after about a week.

Anyone who has been through an episode of food poisoning understands how absolutely miserable it is. Prevention is best, so cooking meats to their proper temperature and washing produce to remove any offending pathogens are essential. If the bacteria find their way into a person's intestinal system, however, consuming coconut oil can decrease the severity or duration of the illness. Coconut oil has demonstrated antibacterial activity against *E. coli* in several studies through its medium-chain fatty acids. Up to 80 percent of *E. coli* was destroyed when exposed to a concentrated source of medium-chain fatty acids from coconut oil,[37] mostly due to lauric acid, but monolaurin, the derivative of lauric acid in the body, was also found to be effective.[38] Coconut oil's capric acid makes monocaprin in the body. Monocaprin is able to reduce viable bacterial counts by up to 99.99 percent in ten minutes in the lab.[39] These compounds work by destroying the bacterial cell membrane, leaking its cytoplasmic contents, and causing cell death. Coconut oil is an effective, natural, and safe product that can eliminate *E. coli* in the body and reduce the symptoms of illness.

18. GASTRIC CANCER

Gastric cancer is stomach cancer. The cells in the lining of the stomach begin to grow uncontrollably and can spread to nearby organs or to the lymph vessels and nodes, where the cancer can be carried to other parts of the body. It grows slowly and tends to only show symptoms in later stages. Stomach cancer is more common in men than women and in those older than their midsixties. The nitrites and nitrates in processed meats have been shown to cause stomach cancer in lab animals, so skipping the pepperoni on pizza or the bacon with eggs is a good idea. Smoking can double the risk of stomach cancer, and secondhand smoke is just as dangerous. A third common cause of stomach cancer is infection with *Helicobacter pylori* (*H. pylori*) bacteria. Most people with this infection never develop stomach cancer, but long-term infection can cause inflammation of the inner lining of the stomach, giving rise to precancerous changes. Symptoms can include nausea, vomiting, loss of appetite, sensation of feeling full, abdominal pain, and heartburn. Conventional treatments include medications, surgery, chemotherapy, and radiation.

Coconut oil can help alleviate pain[40] associated with stomach cancer and can be used to reduce the risk of developing this cancer from *H. pylori*. Monocaprin and monolaurin, derivatives of fatty acids in coconut oil, showed high activity against *H. pylori*.[41] They work by dissolving the lipid membrane of the bacteria, preventing them from replicating and inducing cell death. Lauric acid was also very effective in destroying these bacteria, and when combined with monolaurin and monocaprin, the effect was additive.[42] Replacing a portion of other fats in the diet with coconut oil and consuming a ketogenic diet can increase the availability of ketones in the body. The liver can convert coconut oil's medium-chain fatty acids into ketones, which can then be used as an alternate fuel source for the body instead of glucose. Most tumor cells, on the other hand, only use glucose as their fuel source. Providing ketones as an alternative effectively starves cancer cells and allows normal cells to survive. Not all cancers behave this way, so it's important to talk to your doctor before deciding on a ketogenic diet for therapeutic purposes.

19. GINGIVITIS

Gingiva is the part of the gum around the base of the teeth that can become diseased and result in gingivitis. The gums tend to bleed easily, become puffy, and turn from pink to red. They begin to recede, and tooth decay sets in. Gingivitis is caused when hardened plaque, called tartar, forms below and above the gum line. Tartar is full of bacteria, and it is the bacteria that begin the infection. Plaque is formed daily on the teeth, but it can easily be removed through daily brushing and flossing. If it is left to harden into tartar, it is much harder to eliminate. This disease is common, and symptoms are often so mild that most people don't know they have it. Professional teeth cleaning is needed, followed by a good oral hygiene routine at home.

An effective preventative for gingivitis is to use coconut oil pulling. Put a tablespoon of coconut oil in the mouth and allow it to melt. Gently swish in and around the teeth, over the tongue, and along the gums for about fifteen minutes. The medium-chain fatty acids in the oil have antibacterial properties and are able to destroy the bacteria in the mouth that cause the plaque leading to gingivitis. They disrupt the bacterial cell membranes, resulting in cell death. One study in teenage children introduced coconut oil pulling into their daily oral hygiene routine. After seven days, significant reductions in plaque and gingivitis symptoms were noted, with results continuing to improve over the thirty-day experiment.[43] Coconut oil pulling should be done every day if gingivitis is present or up to three times a week in healthy gum tissue for preventative measures.

20. GONORRHEA

Gonorrhea is a sexually transmitted bacterial disease that affects the mucous membranes of the reproductive tract, mouth, throat, eyes, and rectum. Although it is usually transmitted by sex, a baby can get it from its mother during birth. In these cases, the baby's eyes are usually affected. Often, those infected with gonorrhea do not display any symptoms. Some men do experience painful

NUTRITION

HEALTH

WELL-BEING

BEAUTY

urination, penile discharge, or testicle pain. In women, symptoms include painful urination and intercourse, increased vaginal discharge, and abnormal vaginal bleeding. An infected rectum may be itchy and sore with painful bowel movements. Throat infections can cause sore and swollen tissue. Whether gonorrhea shows symptoms or not, untreated cases can lead to infertility, increased risk of HIV, or a life-threatening condition called disseminated gonococcal infection. Fortunately, gonorrhea can be treated with antibiotics. Unfortunately, strains of drug-resistant gonorrhea are emerging, making the successful treatment of gonorrhea increasingly more difficult.

Because of antimicrobial resistance, an alternative treatment for gonorrhea is crucial. Research has uncovered the potency of several medium-chain fatty acids and their derivatives that are able to quickly and powerfully inactivate different strains of gonorrhea bacteria. In one study, lauric acid and monocaprin were highly effective in killing all five strains of gonorrhea tested in just one minute of exposure. Under the same conditions, capric acid and monolaurin eliminated some of the strains completely and others partially.[44] Both lauric acid and capric acid are found in coconut oil. Monocaprin and monolaurin are formed from these fatty acids in the body. They all work by destroying the cell membranes of gonorrhea bacteria, leading to cell death. Because coconut oil contains these antibacterial fatty acids, applying it topically to the rectum, to the genitals, around the eyes, or as a gargling agent for infections of the throat should help reduce or eliminate the infection. If taken preventatively, any infection from future contact with gonorrhea bacteria should be deterred.

21. HAEMOPHILUS INFLUENZA

Unlike its name suggests, *Haemophilus influenzae* is not related to the flu. It is a bacterial infection that mostly affects babies and young children, although people of all ages are susceptible. There are many strains of these bacteria, and they can cause a wide variety of conditions and diseases from mild earaches to severe blood infections. People are most familiar with *Haemophilus influenzae* strain b, or Hib, that can cause meningitis. Hib can be prevented with a vaccine, but this vaccine only protects against Hib and not against any of the other *Haemophilus influenzae* strains. These other strains can cause lung, skin, blood, ear, eye, or nasal infections and infect the joints, bones, or the nervous system. They are spread when an infected person sneezes, coughs, or talks, sending respiratory droplets containing the bacteria out into the air. Nearby people inhale this air, and the bacteria enter their respiratory system. They nestle into the respiratory lining or enter the bloodstream where they are carried to other organs in the body. Treatment often involves specific antibiotics, but these can increase the risk of infection or blood clots.

The numerous strains and variety of infections *Haemophilus influenzae* cause make it challenging to find an effective multistrain treatment that is safe and nontoxic. In addition, *Haemophilus influenzae* exhibits widespread antibiotic resistance, so the need for alternative therapies is increasingly important. Coconut oil is made up of almost 50 percent lauric acid. This has antibacterial activity and also converts to monolaurin in the body, which is even more potent than lauric acid in killing bacteria. Monolaurin is able to inactivate *Haemophilus influenzae* by disintegrating its bacterial cell membrane. An added benefit is that monolaurin doesn't appear to destroy the good bacteria in the gut like conventional antibiotics.[45] Consuming coconut oil can aid the immune system in eliminating *Haemophilus influenzae* from the body. For skin, eye, or ear infections, topical application can be used to speed recovery and alleviate symptoms. Apply directly to the infected area several times a day.

22. HEPATITIS C

Hepatitis C is a viral disease that affects the liver. It is contracted through contaminated blood and can live in the body for many years before symptoms begin to appear. Most people do not know they have hepatitis C until the virus begins to damage the liver and symptoms develop like fever, nausea, diarrhea, poor appetite, fatigue, jaundice, muscle aches, and bleeding issues. If left untreated, hepatitis C can cause scarring of the liver—which impairs its function—liver cancer, or even liver failure. Without the liver, the body cannot survive. In earlier stages, hepatitis C can be treated with antiviral medications to clear the virus from the system. If the liver is too damaged or low functioning, a liver transplant may be required.

Coconut oil contains many fatty acids that are capable of destroying viruses that have lipid membranes like the hepatitis C virus.[46] They break apart the lipid membrane by dissolving the lipids, causing cell death. One of the products formed in the body from coconut oil is monolaurin. This fatty acid is thought to interrupt the signal the virus sends to the host cell.[47] The virus can no longer bind with the host and replicate. Another fatty acid in coconut oil, linoleic

NUTRITION

HEALTH

WELL-BEING

BEAUTY

acid, inhibits hepatitis C from replicating.[48] Without the ability to produce new viral material, the disease becomes self-limiting and will eventually cease. Coconut oil can be consumed on a daily basis to provide the necessary fatty acids to fight hepatitis C and complement medicinal treatments like interferon therapy, which boosts the body's immune system.

23. HIV

HIV or human immunodeficiency virus is a sexually transmitted disease that can be spread through bodily fluids from one infected person to another or from mother to child during pregnancy, birth, or breastfeeding. HIV attacks the body's immune system and destroys cells the body uses to fight off infections and disease. Opportunistic infections and cancers can develop and spread unabated. There are three stages of the disease. The first stage can last for several weeks, and those infected may experience fever, headache, sore throat, and muscle pain. The second stage often has no symptoms, and if antiretroviral medications are taken, the progression can be slowed for decades. Without treatment, the immune system gets badly damaged, and within a decade, the disease progresses to stage three, known as AIDS or acquired immunodeficiency syndrome. The body is susceptible to many infections at this stage, and survival time dramatically decreases. Once HIV is detected, treatment with a combination of anti-HIV drugs should begin to keep viral levels low. Unfortunately, there is no cure for HIV.

When coconut oil is ingested, capric acid is converted into monocaprin. This compound was studied for its potential against sexually transmitted diseases. Monocaprin was dissolved in a hydrogel and mixed with human semen infected with HIV in a laboratory setting. After one minute, HIV was inactivated ten thousandfold.[49] Other fatty acids in coconut oil like lauric acid are also effective against a variety of viruses and could target HIV.[50] A study using monolaurin or coconut oil for six months in fifteen untreated HIV patients found that consuming either monolaurin capsules or 45 milliliters (3 tablespoons) of coconut oil a day decreased viral load.[51] This study is supported by documented cases of HIV/AIDS patients decreasing their viral load to nearly undetectable levels by consuming 3 1/2 tablespoons of coconut oil or half a coconut a day.[52] Coconut oil must be ingested for monocaprin and monolaurin to be produced by the body. Daily consumption would provide these compounds to assist in the fight against HIV and reduce viral load.

24. HYPERLIPIDEMIA

This is a condition in which there are high levels of fat in the blood, like cholesterol and triglycerides. Hyperlipidemia causes atherosclerosis,[53] a disease in which plaque builds up inside the arteries, the blood vessels that carry oxygen-rich blood to the body. Plaque collects along the arterial walls and is made up of fat, cholesterol, calcium, and other substances. Over time, it hardens and makes the arterial path smaller. If not treated, blood flow can become so constricted that a heart attack, stroke, or even death may result. Atherosclerosis is a very common disease and often exists without any outward symptoms. The risk factors include an unhealthy diet, lack of exercise, and smoking. It is not surprising, then, that the main treatment is a change in lifestyle to incorporate healthy choices.

Coconut oil is effective in reducing high blood fat levels. A study of Filipino women found that consuming coconut oil was positively associated with HDL (good) cholesterol and did not have an impact on LDL (bad) cholesterol or triglycerides.[54] Having elevated levels of HDL cholesterol is important because they pick up the LDL cholesterol and bring it to the liver, reducing levels in the blood. LDL cholesterol can become oxidized by free radicals, which activate the inflammatory response in the arterial walls and lead to the development of plaque. The medium-chain fatty acids in coconut oil, particularly the abundant lauric acid, can increase antioxidant activity[55] and neutralize free radicals so they cannot oxidize LDL cholesterol. Coconut oil also contains polyphenols, which are antioxidants themselves. Their actions prevent arterial tissue damage. Another study in women over a twelve-week period showed that dietary consumption of 30 milliliters (2 tablespoons) of coconut oil increased HDL cholesterol levels and lowered the ratio of LDL to HDL cholesterol. Other participants in the study received soybean oil and had higher total cholesterol, higher LDL cholesterol, and a higher LDL to HDL ratio.[56] All these factors indicate coconut oil is superior to soybean oil in terms of influence on blood lipids and has a cardioprotective effect. It can lower undesirable fats and elevate beneficial fats in the blood. Consuming 2 tablespoons of coconut oil a day can be done in place of consumption of other vegetable oils to reduce the risk of heart disease.

NUTRITION

HEALTH

WELL-BEING

BEAUTY

25. HYPERTENSION

The force exerted against arterial walls as blood flows through them determines blood pressure. The pressure is measured in the arteries when the heart contracts (systolic) and when the heart is at rest (diastolic). It is determined by how much blood the heart pumps and the resistance it encounters as it flows through the arteries. Blood pressure sustained above 140/90 mmhg (millimeters of mercury) is considered high and is called hypertension. This condition develops slowly over time, and many people have it without knowing. It can damage blood vessels and the heart. If left untreated, it can lead to heart attack and stroke. Primary hypertension doesn't have any identifiable cause, although obesity, smoking, poor diet, lack of exercise, and high salt intake are some common risk factors. Secondary hypertension has an underlying cause and could result from drugs or certain medications, alcohol abuse, thyroid problems, or kidney issues. Hypertension responds well to changes in lifestyle. Exercising more, eating a nutrient-rich diet, reducing stress, and quitting smoking and alcohol consumption should bring blood pressure down. There are many drugs available to lower blood pressure, including thiazide diuretics to reduce blood volume, beta blockers to slow down the heart rate, ACE inhibitors to block the action of some hormones that regulate blood pressure, and calcium channel blockers and renin inhibitors to widen the arteries. All these medications come with significant side effects like diarrhea, fatigue, dizziness, nausea, erectile dysfunction, and headaches.

Changes in lifestyle should be the first line of defense against high blood pressure. If additional measures are needed, try including 2 tablespoons of coconut oil in the diet each day before relying on any of the medications described above. Blood pressure could be lowered without having to endure any of the many side effects of conventional drugs. A recent study determined that including coconut oil in the diet for thirty days reduces arterial blood pressure in hypertensive rats compared to hypertensive rats fed saline in place of coconut oil.[57] In humans, an interesting observation of coconut oil consumption was noted in Sri Lanka between 1978 and 1991. The number of coconuts in the diet decreased by 25 percent and were replaced with corn oil and other vegetable oils. As coconut oil consumption declined, heart disease increased.[58] Because hypertension is a risk factor for heart disease, consuming coconut oil should lower blood pressure and reduce this risk.

26. LEUKEMIA

Leukemia is a cancer of the body's blood-forming tissues. Adult T-cell leukemia affects the immune system's T-cells that destroy germs and cancer cells. This disease is caused by a T-cell leukemia virus and is transmitted sexually, through blood transfusions or through breastfeeding. It may lie dormant in the body for decades, but when it becomes active, it is rapidly fatal. This is because the virus is poorly impacted by cancer drugs and because once active, T-cell functions become severely impaired, leaving the body open to opportunistic infections. Less than 5 percent of individuals with the virus develop adult T-cell leukemia, and there is no way of predicting in which infected individuals this may occur. Those that do develop the leukemia suffer from enlarged lymph nodes, spleen, and liver as well as skin and bone lesions, fever, fatigue, and a host of other symptoms. Because this disease is so rare, there are no established treatment standards in the United States. Therapy includes a combination of chemotherapy drugs. Sometimes, stem cell transplants are given to those in remission to replace diseased bone marrow with healthy tissue.

Coconut oil boosts the immune system and can greatly benefit leukemia patients by helping to provide protection against infections. The medium-chain fatty acids are antimicrobial and have the ability to fight bacteria, viruses, fungi, and parasites. By attacking any of these invading organisms, the immune system can spend its energy fighting the leukemia virus. Coconut oil could also be effective in destroying the leukemia virus itself. The fatty acids and their derivatives are known to have the ability to break down protective lipid membranes like the membrane of the leukemia virus.[59]

27. LIPODYSTROPHY

The abnormal and progressive loss of fat tissue under the skin or around internal organs is called lipodystrophy. This fat loss can occur all over the body or in just one particular area and gives the appearance of dents or sunken areas under the skin. In some cases, when fat is lost in one area, it is accumulated in another. Small lumps or larger humps result. This condition is associated with metabolic abnormalities like insulin resistance, diabetes, high blood fat levels, and fatty liver disease. It is rare and affects mostly children and young adults, particularly females. The onset of fat loss is slow and usually involves the disappearance of fat under the skin of the face, neck, and upper body. In females, fat often accumulates in the buttocks and lower limbs, but this does not usually happen in males. Lipodystrophy is a nonfatal condition but is associated with the onset of kidney failure and pregnancy complications. At this point, there are no known treatments to slow or prevent fat tissue loss and redistribution.

When this condition causes sunken areas of the skin, coconut oil can be used to fill the site so that the skin appears smooth and even. One doctor treated a patient with lipodystrophy that had deep depressions in the front of her thighs from insulin injections. The doctor boiled coconut oil and injected it into the depression once the oil had cooled enough to be tolerable. Results were immediately noticeable. Over the next eight years, the improvement gradually declined, and after the woman gained a considerable amount of weight, the depression was pronounced once again. Two more injections were given, one in each leg. The left thigh was injected with coconut oil, as before, which improved appearance with only a slight depression after four months. The right thigh was injected with coconut oil and Parowax. After four months, the results on this leg were even better and the depression was gone.[60] Coconut oil can be used as a nontoxic filler under the skin. Note, though, that this procedure should only be done by a medical professional.

NUTRITION

HEALTH

WELL-BEING

BEAUTY

28. LISTERIOSIS

Listeriosis is a serious infection caused by eating food contaminated with the bacteria *Listeria monocytogenes*. These bacteria are contracted by humans most commonly through deli meats, hot dogs, unpasteurized milk, and soft cheeses. Most people who come into contact with these bacteria are not seriously affected and may experience muscle aches, headaches, nausea, and diarrhea. Pregnant mothers need to be very vigilant during pregnancy because *Listeria* can be life threatening to the fetus and newborn baby. People with weakened immune systems are also at higher risk of developing serious or life-threatening complications. This illness usually runs its course without intervention, but in high-risk patients, antibiotics are commonly prescribed.

Coconut oil can be consumed as a preventative to listeriosis and can even be sprayed on paper towels (in liquid form) and wrapped around soft cheeses, hot dogs, and deli meats to prevent the growth of the bacteria. Research was performed on the ability of either lauric acid—coconut oil's most abundant fatty acid—or nisin, a common preservative in processed foods, to inhibit the growth of *Listeria monocytogenes*. The compounds were added to biofilm and tested in both a liquid medium and on turkey bologna infected with *Listeria monocytogenes*. Biofilm with lauric acid and nisin together reduced *Listeria* cultures to undetectable levels after eight hours while biofilms with lauric acid alone reduced counts on turkey bologna by ten times after twenty-one days.[61] Lauric acid appears to be very effective in destroying *Listeria* bacteria and can reduce the risk of infection by destroying the bacteria either on food or in the body.

29. LIVER DISEASE

The liver is the largest internal organ in the body. It filters toxins out of the bloodstream to prevent them from damaging tissues. When the liver tissue itself becomes damaged, it has the ability to regenerate and make new, healthy tissue. When the damage gets too extensive, however, liver disease sets in and the liver no longer functions as it should. A number of conditions can cause liver disease, including hepatitis A, B, and C, cirrhosis of the liver, nonalcoholic fatty liver disease, and alcoholic hepatitis. Symptoms include abdominal swelling and pain, bruising, fatigue, loss of appetite, and jaundice. Lifestyle modifications are recommended depending on the specific cause of the disease. Eliminating alcohol, losing weight, taking medications, or undergoing surgery help reverse or slow progression. If damage is too severe, liver transplants may be necessary.

A study published using laboratory rats showed pretreatment with virgin coconut oil significantly reduced the extent of liver damage induced by the administration of 3 grams/kilogram of the pain reliever acetaminophen. Through the study, liver weight was not significantly increased, and the viability of liver cells was maintained compared to controls.[62] Coconut oil may also help prevent or treat nonalcoholic fatty liver disease, which is becoming more prevalent today with the rise in diabetes. It provides this protective effect by targeting the factors that contribute to the condition. It has phenolic compounds that are potent antioxidants[63, 64] that can reduce oxidative stress on the liver as well as anti-inflammatory properties[65] to inhibit inflammation. The antioxidant ability of coconut oil[66, 67] can also guard against alcohol-induced liver damage.

Coconut oil, then, has the potential to be used as a natural supplement for the prevention and treatment of liver disease.

30. MALARIA

Malaria is a serious disease caused by a parasite and is transmitted by mosquitoes. Over 200 million people were infected with malaria in 2015,[68] mostly in tropical and subtropical climates. The United States sees about 1500 reported cases each year, usually from immigrants or travelers returning from tropical countries. This disease can be fatal, and many experience high fever, quivering chills, and flulike symptoms. About 90 percent of fatalities occur in Africa from complications that develop as the disease progresses. Unfortunately, young children succumb most often.

Once bitten, it takes several weeks or as long as a year for symptoms to appear. Some varieties of the disease can cause relapses after the initial episode of illness. The parasite lays dormant for months or years and then reactivates. If malaria is diagnosed and treated in the early stages, it is curable. Caution is warranted when traveling to countries where malaria is prevalent. Taking antimalarial drugs before, during, and after the trip can kill the parasite and prevent the onset of symptoms. However, many of the parasites are now immune to antimalarial drugs, and a constant search for new therapeutics is ongoing.

Folk medicine has a long and colorful history that sheds light on ancient treatments and cures for a variety of illnesses. In Malaysia, coconuts have traditionally been used as a remedy for malaria. To test the credibility of using coconuts therapeutically, an extract of the coconut flesh containing the oil was administered to malaria-infected mice. A significant reduction in the parasite was noted, although survival time in the infected mice was not increased. Despite this, the pharmacological constituents of coconut oil, notably the polyphenols, have demonstrated antimalarial activity,[69] and further work into developing a therapeutic agent using coconut oil is validated.

31. MEASLES

Measles is a very contagious disease caused by a virus that replicates in the nose and throat. This virus can become airborne and is spread from an infected person by coughing, sneezing, or sharing food or drink. The virus can remain active on surfaces for several hours, so washing hands frequently around symptomatic individuals is recommended. Infections begin like a bad cold—high fever, sore throat, runny nose, cough—but worsen with the onset of diarrhea and sore, red eyes. These symptoms subside, and a red rash appears all over the body. The contagious period extends from four days before the onset of the rash to four days after. This disease is relatively rare in North America today because most children are vaccinated against it when they are very young. If contracted, a post-exposure vaccination or an injection of antibodies can be given within a certain time frame to lessen the severity of the illness. Once firmly established, however, measles has to run its course.

Measles is a lipid-coated virus, meaning it has a protective layer around its genetic material made up of fats and other compounds. Coconut oil has been found to be very effective in destroying lipid-coated viruses[70] like the measles virus. It does this through monolaurin, which is converted from lauric acid, the most abundant fatty acid in coconut oil. Monolaurin solubilizes lipids in the protective membrane of the virus and interrupts the signal that allows the virus to bind to the host cell.[71] If the measles virus cannot bind with the host cell, it is unable to inject its genetic material into the host cell for replication, effectively preventing the virus from spreading. As a precaution, if exposed to anyone with measles, consume between 2 teaspoons (for children) and 3 tablespoons (for adults) of virgin coconut oil a day. This should help destroy the viral infection and prevent or reduce the severity of the symptoms.

32. METABOLIC SYNDROME

Metabolic syndrome is not a disease but rather a group of risk factors that can occur together and collectively raise the possibility of heart disease, stroke, and diabetes. There are five risk factors: a large waistline, a high triglyceride level, a low HDL (good) cholesterol level, high blood pressure, and high fasting blood sugar levels (or insulin resistance). At least three of these factors have to be present for a person to be diagnosed with metabolic syndrome. Because this syndrome is closely associated with obesity and a lack of exercise, changes in dietary and physical habits should significantly improve all risk factors. These changes require a lifelong commitment to healthy living and are the preferred way to improve the body's metabolic functioning. To assist the process, doctors may suggest medications to help control blood pressure, cholesterol, and blood glucose levels.

Medium-chain fatty acids are instrumental in improving blood lipid profiles that can lead to heart disease. A study of Filipino women found that consuming coconut oil was positively associated with HDL cholesterol levels and did not have an impact on the triglycerides.[72] Many other fats and oils raise triglycerides levels. Another study in women over a twelve-week period showed that daily dietary consumption of 30 milliliters (2 tablespoons) of coconut oil increased HDL cholesterol levels and lowered the ratio of LDL (bad) to HDL cholesterol.[73]

High blood pressure can also be improved by adding coconut oil to the diet. A recent study found that hypertensive rats consuming coconut oil for thirty days reduced arterial blood pressure compared to hypertensive rats fed saline instead.[74] A correlation exists in humans as well. In Sri Lanka between 1978 and 1991, coconut consumption decreased by 25 percent and was replaced with corn oil and other vegetable oils. As coconut oil consumption declined, heart disease increased.[75]

Medium-chain fatty acids like those found in coconut oil are known to increase metabolism and promote weight loss. Because of their size, medium-chain fatty acids are absorbed directly from the intestines and are delivered to the liver, oxidized, and used for energy. They do not get readily stored in fat cells like the long-chain fatty acids found in many fats, like olive oil and soybean oil. This positive effect on body weight was demonstrated by a study following twenty obese human volunteers who consumed virgin coconut oil during a four-week period. At the conclusion of the study, waist circumference was significantly reduced from starting measurements.[76] These results confirmed an earlier study on women that found consuming coconut oil reduced not only abdominal fat but also their body mass index.[77] Reducing abdominal fat decreases one of the risk factors for metabolic syndrome.

Coconut oil can even improve blood glucose levels. In diabetic male rats fed coconut oil once a day over four weeks, fasting blood glucose levels were significantly reduced and serum insulin levels increased.[78] This hypoglycemic action of coconut oil can help manage high blood sugar levels and can be used as an alternative to medication to reduce the risk of developing diabetes in nondiabetic individuals.

Taken together, coconut oil can help control all five risk factors of metabolic syndrome. Depending on the severity of symptoms, up to 3 tablespoons of virgin coconut oil can be consumed each day, along with a healthy diet and exercise.

33. MONONUCLEOSIS

Otherwise known as mono or the "kissing disease," mononucleosis is a contagious viral infection, usually caused by the Epstein-Barr virus. It is very common and affects mostly teenagers and young adults. Contact through saliva, mucus of the nose and throat, or even tears can transmit the virus from an infected person to a healthy person, so avoid kissing or sharing toothbrushes, utensils, or food with someone carrying the virus. Mono can bring fatigue, a sore throat, fever, a headache, swollen lymph nodes, a skin rash, or a swollen spleen. Rest, fluids, and a healthy diet are recommended to help the body fight the infection. It usually goes away on its own and is not very serious, although complications involving the spleen and liver can be severe.

The Epstein-Barr virus silently multiplies in the body for four to six weeks before symptoms begin, and then the infection continues for another few weeks to months. Being able to reduce the viral load in the body should lessen the duration and severity of symptoms, a very desirable outcome for infected individuals. Medium-chain fatty acids, found in abundance in coconut oil, prevent Epstein-Barr viral reproduction by inhibiting the virus from destroying its host cell membrane so that it can no longer spread the virus to other areas to seek new host cells for further replication.[79] This limits the infection to a nonreplicating population of viruses that will be cleared by the immune system, putting an end to the infection. Consuming up to 3 tablespoons of coconut oil each day will provide the medium-chain fatty acids needed to alleviate mononucleosis symptoms and prevent its spread to others.

34. OSTEOPOROSIS

Osteoporosis is a bone disease in which the body can't produce enough new bone to replace old bone removal. The process of bone absorption and replacement happens continuously in the body and, in those with osteoporosis, bone mass decreases over time. A decrease in mass and density results in weakened bones that are more likely to break. It is more common in women than men because women have lower bone masses. Osteoporosis is known as a silent disease because it doesn't produce symptoms and diagnosis is often made after a bone has been broken. This disease does run in families, so if a parent or grandparent had osteoporosis, there is an increased chance the next generation will have it too. Certain diseases and medications can also increase the likelihood of developing osteoporosis. A healthy diet sufficient in bone-producing minerals, weight-bearing exercises, and medication are recommended for management and treatment.

Oxidative stress is thought to play a role in the onset of osteoporosis. Two factors associated with high levels of oxidative stress in the body are hypertension and diabetes.[80] Coconut oil has been shown to decrease blood pressure[81] and lower high blood sugar levels.[82] Because oxidative stress reduces bone formation,[83] an increase in antioxidant enzymes to attenuate reactive oxygen molecules will prevent bones from deteriorating. Virgin coconut oil increases antioxidant levels in the body and can prevent bone loss by stopping the damage caused by oxidation. This is particularly important in women, as estrogen levels drop after menopause and, with it, the protective effects estrogen has on the body's oxidative stress. Menopausal rats given virgin coconut oil in their diet for six weeks increased their antioxidant levels compared to control rats who were not fed coconut oil.[84] A similar protocol study showed menopausal rats supplemented with virgin coconut oil had significantly greater bone volume and spongy bone tissue than control rats.[85] Daily consumption of coconut oil should reduce the risk of osteoporosis by minimizing oxidative stress in the body.

35. PANCREATITIS

The pancreas is a large gland situated behind the stomach, next to the small intestine. It is extremely important in digestion and releases powerful enzymes into the small intestine to break down food. Pancreatitis results when the digestive enzymes are activated before they are released into the small intestine. They attack the pancreas, causing inflammation and damage. Acute pancreatitis occurs suddenly and lasts only a few days. Common symptoms are upper abdominal pain that may radiate to the back or increase after eating, tender abdomen, rapid pulse, nausea, vomiting, and fever. Chronic pancreatitis describes long-lasting inflammation of the pancreas. The symptoms are the same as acute pancreatitis but also include weight loss and oily stools. Most cases are caused by long-term alcohol use, but gallstones, medications, high triglycerides, trauma, or genetics are some other contributing factors. Pain is severe with this disease, and pain medications are typically prescribed. Sometimes, pancreatic enzymes are given and a low-fat diet is recommended. If the disease is serious, surgery to remove the gallbladder, damaged pancreatic tissue, or bile duct obstructions is done, if warranted.

It is difficult to manage pancreatic pain that develops after a meal. The medium-chain fatty acids in coconut oil, which exist in abundance, can be used for this purpose. In patients with chronic pancreatitis, feeding a formulation containing medium-chain fatty acids and hydrolyzed peptides—protein broken down into smaller pieces—over a ten-week period improved pain by almost 62 percent. At the same time, the pancreatic output of digestive enzymes was greatly diminished, unburdening the pancreas from this important function.[86] Coconut oil is absorbed directly through the intestinal wall without having to be broken down further by enzymes like long-chain fatty acids. Consuming coconut oil in place of other fatty acids that have long chains—meats, dairy, seeds, nuts, and many vegetable oils—can reduce the workload of the pancreas and ease pain after eating. The pancreas can begin to heal, improving inflammation and restoring optimal function.

NUTRITION

HEALTH

WELL-BEING

BEAUTY

NUTRITION

HEALTH

WELL-BEING

BEAUTY

36. RINGWORM

Worms do not actually cause this condition. Ringworm is a fungal infection of the outer layers of skin that is characterized by a red rash that forms a circle, or ring, on the surface of the skin with a clearer patch of skin in the middle. The fungus can affect any area of the body with one or many rings. It is contagious and is spread from one infected person or animal to another. Even touching bedding, towels, or surfaces that were in contact with the fungus can cause it to adhere to the skin and begin to multiply. Children are most susceptible. Initially, the rash is red, itchy, and flat. If it progresses, the skin can become inflamed with pus-filled blisters. Over-the-counter fungal creams can be used to get rid of the infection, but in severe cases, prescription antifungal medications may be needed.

A popular home remedy to treat the fungus causing ringworm is coconut oil. The medium-chain fatty acids in the oil are potent antifungal agents.[87] Lauric acid, the most abundant fatty acid, and monolaurin, derived from lauric acid in the body, are reported to inactivate or kill several species of ringworm.[88] However, these aren't the only constituents coconut oil has to offer in the fight. Its polyphenol compounds are also effective antifungals. Extracts of polyphenols from other plant sources were tested on two ringworm species, and the growth of both populations were inhibited.[89] At a time when current drug therapy is limited and often ineffective, using coconut oil as a natural, safe, and effective treatment can offer affordable and accessible relief. Coconut oil can be massaged directly onto the skin over the affected area. Apply several times a day. At night, put a thicker layer over the skin and cover with a wrap. This allows the oil's fatty acids and polyphenols to work all night. The infection should clear within several weeks.

....

37. SALMoNELLOSiS

This is a type of food poisoning caused by the *Salmonella* bacteria. It enters the system through contaminated food. This contamination can happen to poultry, beef, milk, eggs, and even vegetables during food processing and handling. *Salmonella* is also found in some pets, ducklings, reptiles, hamsters, and other small rodents. Hand washing is recommended after handling these animals to prevent infection. If *Salmonella* poisoning does happen, it usually occurs within twelve to seventy-two hours after it enters the body. Diarrhea, stomach cramps, and fever develop and can last up to a week. They eventually subside without medication.

There is no way to know if produce contains the *Salmonella* bacteria because the food looks and smells normal. The best way to avoid infection is by prevention. This can begin with feeding chicks coconut oil to reduce bacterial counts and control the spread to humans. Caprylic acid, making up about 7 percent of coconut oil, was fed to a group of one-day-old chicks in a randomized controlled trial. On days fifteen and eighteen, *Salmonella* organisms in the group fed caprylic acid were significantly lower than the control birds.[90] In addition to caprylic acid, caproic and capric acids (found in coconut oil) were also found to effectively lower *Salmonella* levels by adding these medium-chain fatty acids in their feed. They are thought to work synergistically to suppress the expression of *Salmonella* genes required for invasion and colonization of the chick's internal organs.[91] Those who have egg-laying chickens in their backyard would be wise to add some coconut oil to their feed. Mix a tablespoon of oil with a half cup of grain for a snack they'll love. If someone is so unfortunate as to get food poisoning, however, eating coconut oil can help shorten the duration of the illness. In the lab, monocaprin, derived from capric acid in the body, was shown to reduce *Salmonella* numbers by 99.99 percent after ten minutes of exposure.[92] To alleviate symptoms and shorten the duration, take 1 teaspoon of coconut oil twice a day. If symptoms are severe, take up to 3 tablespoons a day in divided doses.

38. SKIN CANCER

This common form of cancer is the abnormal growth of skin cells resulting from a mutation that allows the cells to grow out of control and form a cancerous mass. It develops most often on the sun-exposed areas of the skin, but it can develop in areas protected from the harmful ultraviolet (UV) radiation of the sun that often causes it. Other factors, such as exposure to toxic chemicals or a weakened immune system, may also be responsible. There are three types. Basal cell carcinoma appears most often on the face and neck and can look like a waxy bump or scar-like lesion. Squamous cell carcinoma is most frequent in areas of the skin exposed to the sun and can look like a red nodule or a flat lesion with a scaly, crusted surface. Melanomas can appear anywhere and are characterized by large, brownish spots with darker speckles or dark lesions on the hands, feet, or mucous membranes. Moles that change in color or size, that bleed, or that have irregular borders may be melanoma. Surgery, radiation, or topical medications are the conventional treatments for skin cancer.

Coconut oil shows promise as an agent to protect against skin cancer. Cancerous human skin cells were treated for forty-eight hours with different concentrations of three fatty acids found in coconut oil—capric, caprylic and caproic acids. All three acids reduced cancer cell viability by up to 90 percent compared to controls. These acids decrease the cancer cell's ability to replicate and influenced cancer cell death.[93] This suggests coconut oil could be effective as a treatment for skin cancer, along with traditional methods. Applying coconut oil topically will expose skin cells to fatty acids and should reduce cancerous cell numbers. As an added bonus, coconut oil is a natural sunscreen and can block up to 20 percent of UV rays,[94] preventing sun damage and reducing the risk of skin cancer.

39. STAPHYLOCOCCUS INFECTION

There are over thirty types of bacterial *Staphylococcus* (staph) infections, but most are caused by *Staphylococcus aureus* (*S. aureus*). These bacteria are responsible for skin infections, pneumonia, food poisoning, blood poisoning, and toxic shock syndrome. Staph skin infections are most common and are usually minor. They look like pimples, blisters, or boils. More severe infections, however, can show red, swollen rashes with pus or drainage. Many people

NUTRITION

HEALTH

WELL-BEING

BEAUTY

carry these bacteria on their skin or in their noses without any symptoms. The bacteria get into the skin through cuts or scrapes, so it is important to keep wounds clean and to wash hands regularly. If the bacteria invade the body and get into the bloodstream, infections can turn up in numerous organs and become life threatening. Treatment for minor staph infections is usually a course of antibiotics or drainage of infected areas. Severe infections require hospitalization. Many varieties of staph have become resistant to antibiotics. New treatments are needed to continue to fight these ubiquitous bacteria.

The beauty of coconut oil is that it contains an abundance of natural antibacterial compounds that work to destroy a variety of microbial species. *S. aureus* is no exception. Up to 90 percent of the bacteria were destroyed when exposed to a concentrated source of medium-chain fatty acids from coconut oil.[95] Most of that activity was due to lauric acid, the most abundant fatty acid in the oil. It is not only lauric acid but its derivative, monolaurin, that proved highly effective against staph. Monolaurin combined with other fatty acids given to rodents with *S. aureus* infections in their nasal passages eradicated up to 83 percent of staph bacteria compared to 50 percent in the group treated with a topical antibiotic.[96] Coconut oil can be considered as an alternative to other traditional oral or topical antibiotics, especially in light of staph's ability to become resistant to many common antibiotics.

40. THYROID FUNCTION

The thyroid is a butterfly-shaped gland situated in the neck above the collarbone. It produces hormones that affect metabolism and control many functions in the body from appetite to growth rate. When normal hormone production of the thyroid is altered, the effects in the body can be far reaching. Underproduction of thyroid hormones causes a condition called hypothyroidism. One of the main symptoms is fatigue, since the body relies on certain levels of these hormones for its energy production. Weight gain, slow heart rate, dry skin, and cold intolerance are also common. Dietary or hormone supplementation may be needed to manage this condition. Overproduction of thyroid hormones is called hyperthyroidism. The excess hormones upset the body's chemical balance and can cause weight loss, insomnia, anxiety, and decreased heat tolerance. Drugs to suppress thyroid function or surgery are used to treat hypothyroidism.

Because the thyroid is central to so many important processes in the body, maintaining optimal functioning is essential to good health. Many of the oils commonly consumed in the North American diet consist of long-chain unsaturated fatty acids. Among these are sunflower oil, olive oil, corn oil, canola oil, and soybean oil. Some of these have their own health benefits, but when it comes to the thyroid, coconut oil acts differently than these oils in a very beneficial way. Unsaturated oils inhibit enzymes from producing thyroid hormones, making the body deficient in progesterone and pregnenolone. These hormones protect the body from stress and help keep us young. Replacing unsaturated fatty acids with coconut oil gives the body a stable oil that is readily metabolized for energy and doesn't interfere with the production of thyroid hormones. This is because coconut oil is mostly made up of saturated medium-chain fatty acids. These acids are not readily oxidized like unsaturated oils, which create free radicals in the body. Free radicals are unstable molecules actively looking for an electron. They

NUTRITION

HEALTH

WELL-BEING

BEAUTY

attack the nearest stable molecule and steal one of their electrons, making that molecule a free radical as well. This begins a chain re-action of creating free radicals that can ultimately destroy the cell. If these are cells of the liver, then the conversion of the thyroid's T4 hormone to the more biologically active T3 hormone is slowed. Using coconut oil can avoid all this stress and damage and keep a normal rate of T4 to T3 hormone conversion. Coconut oil can also help reverse some of the effects of a depressed thyroid. It provides energy to combat fatigue, increases metabolism to aid weight loss, and raises thermal output[97] to warm the body.

41. TRICHOMONIASIS

Trichomoniasis, also known as trich, is a common sexually trans-mitted disease caused by the parasite *Trichomonas vaginalis*. About 3.7 million people in the United States have trich, but only about 30 percent know they have it.[98] Most cases go unnoticed because they are asymptomatic. If symptoms do arise, women can expect a foul-smelling vaginal discharge accompanied by genital itching, painful intercourse, and burning urination. Men may experience itching inside the penis, penile discharge, or a burning sensation during urination or ejaculation. Genital contact with an infected person is needed for contraction of the parasite, and the incuba-tion period is between five and twenty-eight days. Both partners require treatment with antibiotics, followed by abstinence from sexual activity until the infection is gone—usually about a week.

Coconuts have traditionally been used in Mexican medicine to treat trich.[99] It is thought the polyphenols are able to inhibit the growth of the developmental stage of the parasites, causing their death. One study demonstrated the efficacy of pomegranates in completely curing women infected with trich by drinking the juice.[100] Pomegranates, like coconut oil, are sources of polyphenols. If infection with trichomoniasis is suspected or known, consume 1–3 tablespoons of coconut oil a day until the infection has cleared.

42. ULCERS

Ulcers are holes in the protective lining of the stomach, small intestine, and esophagus. Sores develop that may cause stomach pain, bloating, heartburn, nausea, and fatty food intolerance. Infection with *H. pylori* is thought to be the main cause. Overuse of painkillers, smoking, stress, and heavy alcohol use are other contributing factors. If *H. pylori* are present, treatment involves a course of antibiotics to kill the bacteria. Medications to neutralize, block, or reduce the production of stomach acid are often prescribed. It is also imperative that the use of painkillers, smoking, and alcohol use is greatly reduced or stopped.

Some of coconut oil's fatty acids are converted in the body into monolaurin and monocaprin. These acids have been found to be effective against *H. pylori*.[101] Lauric acid, coconut oil's most abundant fatty acid, was also found to destroy *H. pylori* with effectiveness, increasing sharply with decreasing pH. The presence of more than one fatty acid had an additive effect in attenuating the viability of the bacteria.[102] By destroying *H. pylori*, the cause of many ulcers is eliminated.

If excess stomach acid is the origin of ulcers, coconut oil can help here, too. The volume of gastric juice secreted by male rats was significantly reduced after being fed virgin coconut oil. Decreasing stomach acid can reduce the risk of acid damaging the tissue of the stomach and forming painful ulcers. Mucus was also increased, protecting the cells lining the stomach walls.[103] Rather than taking antibiotics or medication to reduce stomach acid production, try consuming a tablespoon of virgin coconut oil each day. This will destroy harmful bacteria, protect the stomach lining, and allow damaged tissue to heal.

43. URINARY TRACT INFECTIONS

Urinary tract infections involve any part of the urinary tract and include the bladder, urethra, kidneys, and ureters. Infections of the bladder are most common. Bacteria in the stool, commonly *E. coli*, can adhere to the skin and make their way into the urethra. Once there, the bacteria move up into the bladder and begin to multiply. Initially, symptoms are not evident, but as the infection progresses, urine output changes. Many report a frequent urge to urinate, burning urination, and urine that smells bad or is cloudy, red, or pink. Pain in the pelvis or abdomen is sometimes seen, and nausea and vomiting can occur. Most urinary tract infections are treated with a course of antibiotics. Sometimes, if the pain or burning sensation is severe, doctors may prescribe pain relievers to numb the bladder and urethra.

Coconut oil is effective in eliminating *E. coli*, the bacteria most commonly responsible for urinary tract infections. Up to 80 percent of the bacteria was destroyed when exposed to a concentrated source of medium-chain fatty acids from coconut oil.[104] This antibacterial activity was mostly due to lauric acid, but monolaurin was also found to be effective.[105] Lauric acid is partially converted to monolaurin in the body, so both compounds are available to work against *E. coli*. In the same way, capric acid makes mono-caprin in the body. Monocaprin is able to reduce viable bacterial counts in ten minutes.[106] They work by disrupting the bacterial cell membranes, which lead to their death. These compounds from co-conut oil don't negatively affect the good intestinal bacteria like antibiotics do, so they are much more beneficial to the body and kinder to the digestive system. As a preventative for urinary tract infections or for use in the early stages, consume 1 tablespoon of coconut oil three times a day. Drink plenty of water to help flush out toxins and speed the healing process.

NUTRITION

HEALTH

WELL-BEING

BEAUTY

CHAPTER 3

MANAGING WELL-BEING

44. ABDOMINAL FAT

The type of fat deposited in the abdominal area is called visceral fat and differs from the fat found under the skin. Visceral fat lies in and around the internal organs and gives the characteristic "beer belly" that causes the stomach to protrude. This type of fat has negative effects on health and is associated with an increased risk of heart disease, diabetes, and some cancers. The main cause for abdominal obesity is simply consuming more calories than the body expends, but genetic and environmental factors like age and hormonal changes may also be contributors. A marker of abdominal obesity is waist circumference. Men with a waist measuring over forty inches and women measuring over thirty-five inches are considered to be abdominally obese and at risk for health complications.

Coconut oil has been found to be effective in reducing abdominal fat. Women presenting with abdominal obesity were supplemented with either soybean oil or coconut oil over a twelve-week period. Their diets were controlled and lower in calories than before enrollment in the study. Participants also walked for fifty minutes each day. At the end of the study, both groups of women had lowered their body mass index, but only the women supplemented with coconut oil reduced their waist circumference. A bonus was that in the coconut oil group, HDL (good) cholesterol levels increased and LDL (bad) cholesterol levels were unaffected. This was not seen in the soybean oil group.[107] It's not just women but also men that benefit. A study of obese men and women supplemented with virgin coconut oil confirmed its effectiveness in reducing waist circumference, with the results being more pronounced in men than women.[108] This effect is likely due to the medium-chain fatty acids in coconut oil. They are absorbed directly from the small intestine and used for energy. Most other commonly consumed fats are made up of long-chain fatty acids and tend to get stored in fat cells.

45. ATHLETE'S FOOT

Wearing sandals in locker rooms and around public pools can help protect feet from a common fungal infection known as athlete's foot. This fungus is highly contagious and can be acquired by sharing shoes, walking on infected surfaces, or directly contacting the skin of an infected foot. Once contracted, the fungus grows on or just under the surface of the skin and thrives in moist, warm places. It's important to dry the feet well, particularly between the toes, to prevent fungus from growing. The fungi can also grow in shoes, so make sure to disinfect all footwear as well.

There are three types of infection. Toe web type occurs between the toes, causing the skin to become itchy, scaly, dry, and cracked. Moccasin type is characterized by a sore foot, followed by thickened skin on the heel or along the bottom of the foot. Vesicular athlete's foot develops as blisters under the skin. Mild infections can be treated with antifungal lotions, but more severe infections may require prescription antifungal topical medications or pills.

Coconut oil contains antifungal fatty acids that can help alleviate the symptoms of athlete's foot by destroying the fungus causing the infection. The same fungus responsible for ringworm causes

NUTRITION

HEALTH

WELL-BEING

BEAUTY

athlete's foot. In one study, several species of ringworm were in-activated or killed by lauric acid, the most abundant fatty acid in coconut oil, and monolaurin, which is derived from lauric acid in the body.[109] These compounds would have the same effectiveness in clearing up athlete's foot. Coconut oil also contains polyphenol compounds that are effective antifungals. Extracts of polyphenols from other plant sources were tested on two ringworm species, and the growth of both populations was inhibited.[110] Apply coco-nut oil liberally to the infected skin and cover with a thin plastic bag. Pull a sock over the bag and leave this treatment on for thirty minutes each day. At night, add a few drops of lavender essential oil to the coconut oil for extra antifungal fighting power that also imparts a soothing scent for bedtime.

46. BRAIN FUNCTION

The brain is the body's command center that receives messages from sensory organs and sends out instructions to the body on how to move and function. It controls everything we do from conscious communication—such as moving muscles, responding to pain, thinking, and reasoning—to the automatic operation of organs and internal processes—like breathing, heart rate, blood pressure, and digestion. The metabolic demand to perform all these tasks is huge, and the brain tells the body to send 20 percent of its oxygenated blood supply to the brain so it can receive oxygen and nutrients as fuel. If fuel sources are inadequate, brain function is compromised. The body fails to work properly, and the mind cannot process all of the countless messages it receives from its billions of nerve cells.

During periods of dieting, low carbohydrate intake, or excessive exercise, the body's reserve of glucose can become depleted. The brain needs an alternate source of energy and is able to use ketones. Medium-chain fatty acids like those in coconut oil are converted into ketones in the liver when glucose stores are used up. The ketones enter the blood and are sent to the brain. Fortunately, they are able to cross the blood-brain barrier. Not all chemicals can. Once inside the brain, they can be used by the cells for energy to drive forward all of its processes. Consuming coconut oil can increase the availability of ketones in the brain during times of glucose depletion. Studies confirm that administration of ketones does elevate levels in the blood[111] and subsequent improvement in cognitive performance.[112, 113]

47. BREAST MILK NUTRITION

Mothers make milk that provides all the necessary nutrients for their babies to grow and thrive. The basic components of milk are fats, proteins, enzymes, vitamins, minerals, and water. Fats in milk are plentiful and are needed as energy for babies to develop their bodies and brains. Breast milk contains lauric acid and capric acid, whose antimicrobial properties protect the baby from infection and disease. In fact, lauric acid and capric acid, both found in abundance in coconut oil, comprise about 20 percent of the saturated fats found in breast milk.

The amount and variety of fatty acids found in breast milk is altered by the mother's diet. Lactating mothers that consume coconut oil significantly increase the amount of lauric acid and capric acid in their breast milk within six hours. The amounts remain elevated for up to twenty-four hours.[114] During this time, the mother passes these compounds on to her baby, who is easily able to digest them due to their relatively small size. These fatty acids can be used immediately to seek out and destroy any invading pathogens and keep baby healthy and strong. Coconut oil is also able to increase the levels of HDL (good) cholesterol and has little effect on LDL (bad) cholesterol. This is especially important in supporting a child's developing immune system; children with infections have been found to have high levels of LDL cholesterol in relation to HDL cholesterol.[115] Adding coconut oil to the mother's diet would provide further protection by decreasing the LDL-to-HDL cholesterol levels. Lactating mothers can safely consume several tablespoons of coconut oil each day. Try this energy-boosting smoothie to get the day started.

COCONUT RASPBERRY SMOOTHIE
ALLRECIPES.COM

2 bananas, broken into chunks
1 cup frozen raspberries
2 tablespoons pecan halves
1 tablespoon coconut oil
1 tablespoon flaxseed meal
1 date, pitted
16 fluid ounces water

1. Place bananas, raspberries, pecans, coconut oil, flax meal, and date in a blender; add water. Blend until smooth.

48. BURNS

A burn causes damage to the skin and possibly underlying tissues from sunlight, heat, chemicals, electricity, or radiation. There are three types of burns. First-degree burns affect the outer layer of skin and cause minor inflammation, redness, and pain. Second-degree burns damage the outer layer of skin and the layer underneath. They are characterized by blisters, redness, and pain. Third-degree burns are the most serious and damage the deepest layer of skin tissue. They have a white, leathery appearance. Treatment for minor burns includes cleaning the wound, applying antibiotic cream, and taking pain medication. More severe burns should be treated by a medical professional.

Coconut oil can be used to replace both the antibiotic cream and the pain medication in the treatment of minor burns. This is a ready and inexpensive remedy that can be prepared at home. Coconut oil contains lauric and capric acids, which reduce inflammation, in part, by inhibiting specific protein complexes and enzymes that trigger it.[116] Reduced swelling alleviates pressure on compressed nerves, so they no longer send pain signals to the brain. The stinging subsides. Coconut oil is also an antibacterial agent and can attack any bacteria that find their way through the damaged skin. This discourages infection and helps the immune system to heal the burn. A study was undertaken in rats comparing the healing rate of burn tissue after application of either coconut oil, a commonly used drug known to prevent infection in burn tissue, or a combination of both. A significant improvement in tissue healing was noted in the coconut-oil-and-drug combination group, and the time to heal was shorter with both coconut oil alone and the combination of coconut oil and the drug compared to controls.[117] For both first- and second-degree burns, apply liberally over the affected tissue and cover with a cloth. Repeat several times a day.

49. CANKER SORES

Canker sores are shallow ulcers that develop on the tongue or inside the lip or cheek. They are round or oval with a red border and yellow or white center. A person may be afflicted with one or many at a time. Cankers can make it hard to eat and talk because they are very painful. The exact cause of cankers is unknown, but several contributing factors common among regular sufferers are stress, hormonal changes, food allergies, acidic food, irritation from braces, biting of the cheek, and nutrient deficiencies. While most minor cankers heal by themselves within several weeks, larger sores can take up to six weeks and can scar the tissue.

A common household remedy for canker sores is coconut oil. The polyphenols in virgin coconut oil are anti-inflammatories and work by decreasing the expression of inflammatory genes in swollen tissue.[118] Lauric acid and capric acid are also able to reduce swelling by inhibiting specific protein complexes and enzymes that trigger inflammation.[119] Reducing the swelling can also help alleviate some of the pain and reduce the risk of biting the area or rubbing braces against it. Virgin coconut oil has been shown to reduce pain[120] and can make movements of the mouth more comfortable, or at least tolerable. The medium-chain fatty acids in coconut oil enhance nutrient absorption,[121, 122] which can help prevent future outbreaks of canker sores, if nutrient deficiency is the cause. Apply a thick layer of solid coconut oil on the sores and try to keep saliva from washing it away for a minute. After this time, swish the melted oil around the mouth a few times and swallow. Do this several times a day. This allows the oil to work directly on reducing the pain and inflammation and should heal the sore within a few days.

50. COLD SORES

Cold sores, or fever blisters, are herpes simplex viral infections that affect the skin around the mouth. Fluid-filled sores develop in and around the lips that eventually break, leaking a clear liquid. A crust then forms. Cold sores tend to group in clusters and are red, swollen, and sore; they can be accompanied by fever and swollen neck glands. Some cold sores last only a few days, while others take weeks to go away. The herpes simplex virus is contagious, and touching the area or sharing utensils, toothbrushes, or razors can spread the infection. The virus gets into the skin through any scratch or tiny cut, so if an outbreak is underway, don't kiss anyone goodnight or share a glass of wine! Once the virus is contracted, it will always be there. It is not always known why an outbreak occurs, but stress and a depressed immune system are thought to be triggers. Treating with antiviral creams, ointments, or pills can reduce symptoms, but these usually only get rid of the cold sores one or two days quicker than without treatment.

When the herpes simplex virus becomes active and results in an outbreak, it not only causes pain and unsightly sores but can

NUTRITION

HEALTH

WELL-BEING

BEAUTY

also be embarrassing for some individuals. That initial tingling sensation associated with an impending outbreak can have a person running for medication or even hiding out until the cold sores have cleared up. Lauric and capric acids in coconut oil are highly effective in killing the herpes simplex virus by tearing apart the viral envelope and causing its contents to leak out. This results in cell death.[123] Lauric acid also inhibits viral reproduction[124] to prevent the spread of infection. Apply coconut oil to the affected area of the mouth several times a day. Try to begin at the first sign of an outbreak to hopefully halt it in its tracks.

51. CONSTIPATION

Constipation is infrequent bowel movements or difficulty in passing stools. It is very common and can be occasional or chronic. Occasional constipation is short term, while chronic constipation is having less than three bowel movements a week for at least three months. Stools move too slowly through the digestive tract, causing them to become hard and dry. They are difficult to pass, and a feeling of not being able to empty the rectum is reported. Increasing fiber intake, fluids, and exercise are known to help increase gastric motility. If that doesn't work, laxatives and other medications to draw water into the intestines are suggested. Side effects of these drugs include bloating, gas, diarrhea, nausea, vomiting, and rectal pain.

Coconut oil provides medium-chain fatty acids that are absorbed into the bloodstream from the intestines and sent to the liver, where they become available to the body's cells for energy. This energy fuels the cell's metabolic processes and boosts overall metabolism. With increased metabolism, a sluggish intestinal digestive process becomes more efficient. Food particles break down and are absorbed at a faster rate. Peristalsis moves the remaining waste through the intestines for elimination. Constipation can also be caused by the presence of too many bad intestinal bacteria and yeasts. These bacteria can overtake the good bacteria that assist in the metabolism of nutrients, intake of vitamins, and absorption of some compounds through the intestinal wall. When good bacterial numbers are low, digestion becomes inefficient and slows down. Slow digestion allows food and waste to remain in the body too long, and constipation may occur. One of the main culprits that overtakes the good bacteria is *Candida*. This common yeast can break down the walls of the intestinal lining, causing inflammation and damage. This affects digestion. Coconut oil is highly effective at destroying *Candida*[125] with capric acid and lauric acid showing the most activity against the yeast. These acids were able to disintegrate the plasma membrane of the yeast and destroy the cells.[126] Coconut oil is also effective at destroying pathogenic bacteria, viruses, and fungi that may inhabit the digestive system and cause problems of constipation. Begin with 1 teaspoon of coconut oil in the morning and 1 teaspoon at night. Gradually increase the amount each time until an effective dose has been reached and bowel movements are regular and easier to pass.

52. DEPRESSION

Depression is a mood disorder that causes a deep sadness and a loss of interest in activities. It affects how a person feels, thinks, and behaves and can cause not just emotional problems but can manifest as physical problems as well. Clinical depression may occur once in a person's lifetime or reoccur multiple times. This feeling of sadness and loss can cause insomnia, loss of appetite, poor concentration, fatigue, suicidal thoughts, and physical symptoms like backaches and headaches. Changes in the body's hormone levels may cause or trigger depression. Modifications of the way brain chemicals work and the effect that has on maintaining stable moods is thought to play a major role. Psychological counseling and antidepressant medications are often prescribed. Antidepressants can cause a wide range of side effects, including nausea, insomnia, blurred vision, weight gain, fatigue, and sexual dysfunction.

Medium-chain fatty acids, which constitute most of coconut oil, have been found to have antidepressant-like effects. After mice showing depressive symptoms were fed these fatty acids, their behavior changed and their depressive symptoms lessened. The acids altered the levels of specific enzymes that are involved in depression and stress.[127] They are also important in combating fatigue associated with depression. They provide a quick yet sustained source of energy, giving the body strength. Increased energy enhances concentration as well. Ketones converted from coconut oil's fatty acids can enter the brain and be used by the cells as fuel to improve mental functioning. This oil is very safe and non-addictive and can be tried as an alternative to the often overused antidepressants.

53. DIAPER RASH

Babies commonly get diaper rash. It appears as red and tender-looking skin in the diaper area—the buttocks, genitals, and thighs. The rash causes discomfort, and the baby may cry or fuss when the area is wiped or washed during baths or diaper changes. Most diaper rashes result from chafing or from the acidity of urine and feces in wet diapers. Sometimes, using new products like ointments, wipes, or laundry detergent can irritate the baby's sensitive skin. Bacterial and yeast infections can spread over this area and produce the characteristic red rash. These pathogens thrive in warm, wet environments. Diaper rash is seen not only in babies but in all people wearing diapers, including adults. Keeping the area clean and dry is the best way to avoid it. Prescription antifungals, antibiotics, and steroid creams can resolve the rash, but each of these present additional issues for the sensitive baby.

Babies have an immature immune system and need protection from bacteria, viruses, fungi, yeasts, and parasites that can affect their health. Chemicals in food and medication should also be avoided. Treating diaper rash with a safe, natural product like coconut oil will benefit babies' rashes without compromising their health. Coconut oil readily penetrates the skin due to its small molecular size and weight, making it a great moisturizer. It has a wonderful soothing effect on chafed skin. If the rash is caused by a fungal infection (likely *Candida*), the fatty acids (particularly lauric and capric acid) in the oil can kill the fungus by destroying its cell membrane.[128, 129] A bacterial skin rash can also be cleared up by coconut oil[130] and eliminate the need for antibiotics. Once again, it's the fatty acids in coconut that can destroy bacteria and eliminate the source of the infection. Try adding a drop of tea tree oil to a teaspoon of coconut oil (warmed to a liquid) for extra fighting power. Apply a thin layer of coconut oil on a clean, dry bottom several times a day.

54. DIARRHEA

Diarrhea describes loose, watery stools. It is very common and usually lasts a few days, although prolonged diarrhea can indicate a medical condition like irritable bowel syndrome. Stomach cramps and pain, bloating, fever, nausea, and vomiting often accompany diarrhea. It occurs when the stool moves too quickly through the colon so the colon doesn't have time to absorb enough liquid from it. The main culprits in causing diarrhea are viruses, bacteria, and parasites. Food intolerance and many medications can also cause diarrhea in susceptible people. If diarrhea persists for more than a few days and if the cause is bacterial or parasitic, doctors may prescribe antibiotics.

Coconut oil has the power to destroy germs in the intestinal system responsible for causing diarrhea. *Campylobacter* bacteria are among the most common infections in humans and can cause bloody diarrhea. A study found monocaprin, derived from capric acid in coconut oil, was very active in killing *Campylobacter*. This same study also tested monocaprin against *Salmonella* and *E. coli*, two other common bacterial infections causing diarrhea in humans. Monocaprin was able to reduce viable bacterial counts in both types of infections.[131] Parasitic infections by *Giardia* are also common in humans worldwide. Lauric acid from coconut oil has been found to be effective in treating giardiasis in hamsters, eliminating up to 82 percent of the parasites.[132] In addition to destroying diarrhea-causing pathogens, coconut oil plays a role in shortening the duration of diarrhea. A study in infants suffering from diarrhea found that a diet of coconut oil, chicken, and plantains ended diarrhea twenty hours faster than a diet of cow's milk.[133] Coconut oil can be used as an effective and natural alternative to more quickly relieve diarrhea with few to no side effects. Begin with 1 teaspoon two times a day and work up to 1 tablespoon twice a day, if needed.

55. DRY EYES

Eyes that burn, sting, or feel scratchy are considered dry eyes. This is a very common condition that affects many people and is caused by a lack of tears. Tears lubricate the surface of the eye and protect it from irritation and infection. They are made up of water, fatty acids, and mucus. Sometimes, the oil gland at the edge of the eyelids becomes blocked, and the composition of tears is low or devoid in fatty acids, resulting in dryness. Evaporation of tears from wind or smoke could also contribute to dry eyes. Mild cases are often relieved by over-the-counter eye drops. If the condition is chronic or more severe, some options include wearing special contact lenses, unblocking oil glands, or taking medications to reduce inflammation and stimulate tears.

It may seem scary to put anything in the eye that doesn't come out of a carefully wrapped and sterilized bottle from the drugstore. That's the route most take to relieve their dry eyes. Those more

NUTRITION

HEALTH

WELL-BEING

BEAUTY

adventurous may want to try coconut oil. Virgin coconut oil was tested for its safety as an eye rewetting agent in rabbits. Drops were instilled three times a day for fourteen days. Data was collected at thirty minutes, sixty minutes, and two weeks. Coconut oil was effective in reducing dry eyes and was found to be completely safe.[134] The fatty acids in coconut oil make it a natural lubricant, while the anti-inflammatory properties of lauric acid and the phenolic acids can reduce redness and itching.

Anything that goes in the eyes should be sterile, and that goes for coconut oil, too. Use a jar of coconut oil specifically for the eyes and be very careful to wash hands before opening the jar. Put a teaspoon of oil into a bowl and place in a larger bowl of warm water. When the oil melts, use a small glass dropper to collect some of the oil and add a drop or two to each eye. Make sure the oil has cooled to a temperature comfortable for the eye. Apply the drops twice a day. Vision will be cloudy at first but quickly clears. The eyes may increase production of natural tears, allowing for the reduced need of the oil.

56. ECZEMA

Eczema is a group of medical conditions that cause the skin to become itchy and inflamed. It is often accompanied by asthma or hay fever and is common in infants (affecting up to 20 percent), although most outgrow eczema by their tenth birthday. It also affects about 3 percent of children and adults who experience it on and off throughout their lives. During a flare-up, the skin is itchy, thickened, dry, and scaly. The skin may be red or brown, and pigmentation could be affected. There are many triggers that cause flare-ups, including scratching, hot showers, stress, clothing, or allergens. Nearly all people with eczema have *Staphylococcus aureus* bacteria on the skin, which multiply rapidly if they penetrate the surface. If this happens, symptoms worsen. Creams and oral drugs to control itching and inflammation can help manage symptoms, and antibiotics can help clear up an infection.

The main goal for treatment of eczema is to relieve itching, since scratching can lead to infection. Coconut oil, applied topically, can do this. The polyphenols in virgin coconut oil are anti-inflammatories and work by decreasing the expression of inflammatory genes in affected tissue.[135] Lauric acid and capric acid are also able to reduce swelling by inhibiting specific protein complexes and enzymes that trigger inflammation.[136] This means the tissue swelling will decrease and no longer press on the nerves that cause itching. If *Staphylococcus aurei* do manage to cause an infection, lauric acid in coconut oil can destroy the bacterial cell.[137] Then the infection should clear. And while lauric acid is highly effective at killing staph skin infections, it does not cause any damage to regular skin cells[138] but, instead, moisturizes the skin and leaves it feeling soothed. Apply a thin layer of coconut oil to the skin several times a day. Repeat as necessary to relieve itching and eliminate infection.

57. ENERGIZE

Everyone has lulls of energy in their day that have them longing for a quick catnap on the couch, but, instead, they often reach for caffeinated beverages to boost their energy and awaken their minds.

A combination of factors can lead to low energy, and common ones are lack of sleep, poor diet, stress, and depression. Taking care to manage the source that drains energy would be a good first step to give bodies what they need to function properly and provide enough energy to happily get through the day. Going to bed earlier, cutting back on saturated fats and sugar, finding outlets to deal with stress, or talking to a therapist are all ways to do this. However, to add even more pep in your step, try taking a little coconut oil every day.

Coconut oil can amp up metabolism by providing an easily digested source of energy. The medium-chain fatty acids, which make up most of the oil, are absorbed directly into the bloodstream, go to the liver, and quickly become available to the cells as fuel. Coconut oil also tries to keep the bad gut bacteria at bay so that the good bacteria can continue to synthesize vitamins and help nutrients be absorbed through the intestinal wall. Both of these are needed for a multitude of metabolic processes in the body. It is not only the body but also the mind that is energized by consuming coconut oil. When glucose stores are low from excessive exercise or dieting, the mind can become sluggish from lack of fuel. During these times, medium-chain fatty acids can be converted into ketones by the liver. These compounds enter the bloodstream and go to the brain, where they can be used as an alternate source of energy. The many metabolic processes happening in the brain can continue without interruption.

If depression is causing fatigue, coconut oil can help here too. The fatty acids have an antidepressant-like effect and work by altering the levels of specific enzymes that are involved in depression and stress.[139] Coconut oil is also very safe and non-addictive, unlike some of the antidepressant medications commonly used. It is an alternative worth considering to energize both the body and the mind.

. . . .

58. FIBROMYALGIA

This disorder is characterized by widespread muscle pain and tenderness. It is thought that the brains of those with fibromyalgia process pain signals differently, amplifying painful sensations. Sleep is often disrupted, fatigue constant, memory impaired, and mood altered. Symptoms can occur gradually over time or be triggered by severe stress, infection, surgery, or trauma. Those suffering from fibromyalgia can take medications for pain or antidepressants to help with sleep. As with any medication, side effects are not uncommon—nausea, rashes, upset stomach, weight gain, and sexual problems are just a few.

Because of their size, the medium-chain fatty acids that make up coconut oil are absorbed from the intestines without being broken into smaller molecules. They are sent to the liver, and from there, they can be directly used as fuel by the cells. This provides a quick and sustained source of energy and can help boost metabolism and alleviate the fatigue felt by many fibromyalgia patients. Pain can be debilitating, but coconut oil can help reduce that pain,[140] which can make the patient feel more comfortable and possibly improve their quality of life. Those that find their memory fading or concentration waning will certainly perk up after consuming coconut oil. The medium-chain fatty acids in the oil can be converted into ketones, which supply the brain with fuel. This can improve cognitive

NUTRITION

HEALTH

WELL-BEING

BEAUTY

function, as was noted in Alzheimer's patients.[141, 142] Having more energy and less pain may be enough to lift the spirits, but coconut oil throws in an added measure to feeling better through its antidepressant-like effect. Medium-chain fatty acids, like those in abundance in coconut oil, were fed to mice showing depressive symptoms. These acids were able to prevent these symptoms by altering the levels of enzymes involved in depression and stress.[143]

59. FLU AND COLDS

Common colds and seasonal flu are respiratory illnesses caused by different viruses. They are highly contagious, and a person can become infected by touching a surface such as a doorknob, stair railing, or bathroom faucet. If the virus gets on the hands and the person then touches their mouth or nose, the virus nestles into the mucosal lining there. Breathing in air near someone who is coughing or sneezing because they are sick with a cold or the flu is another surefire way of getting the virus into the system. There are many different viruses that cause colds and flus. Unless the body has fought the exact virus before, it won't have the right antibodies ready to fight it when it enters the body. The immune system begins an attack against the new virus, and the dreaded symptoms set in. A sore throat, runny or stuffy nose, sneezing, and cough are the hallmarks of a cold. If these symptoms are accompanied by a fever, fatigue, and muscle aches, it is more likely to be the flu. There is no shortage of over-the-counter cold and flu medications, and they are available for every possible symptom. Take a walk down the pharmacy aisle to see antihistamines, decongestants, nasal sprays, cough suppressants, and throat lozenges.

An inexpensive and effective home remedy to combat these symptoms and have you feeling better sooner is coconut oil. Coconut oil contains medium-chain fatty acids that, along with their derivatives, are known antivirals.[144] Most of the activity is attributed to monolaurin, derived from lauric acid in the body. This compound very effectively destroys enveloped coated viruses like the influenza virus, pneumovirus,[145] parainfluenza virus, and the coronavirus. Unfortunately, another common cold virus, the rhinovirus, is non-enveloped and not very susceptible to monolaurin. Monolaurin dissolves the lipids in the viral envelope, causing their outer membrane to fall apart.[146] There is also evidence it interferes with the virus's attempt to communicate with the host cells,[147] preventing entrance into the host cell for replication and maturation. This causes the flu or cold to become self-limiting. Consuming a teaspoon of coconut oil each day can be an effective preventative to colds and flu or to treat an existing cold or flu to shorten the duration and provide relief sooner.

60. GALLSTONES

The gallbladder contains digestive fluid called bile that can crystallize and harden to form gallstones. Most of the stones are made up of cholesterol, but bilirubin—discarded red blood cells—and calcium salts can form stones, too. It is when too much cholesterol or bilirubin is in the bile or when the gallbladder fails to empty properly that gallstones can form. These stones can be as small as a grain of sand or as large as an apricot. Most people with gallstones don't know they have them because they often exhibit no signs or symptoms. If a gallstone blocks a duct, however, there is a sudden

NUTRITION

intense pain in the upper right or center of the stomach, between the shoulder blades, or in the right shoulder. The pain could last from several minutes to a few hours. Doctors treat only gallstones that are causing discomfort. Surgery to remove the entire gallbladder is the recommended choice because gallstone recurrence is frequent. Alternatively, medications can be prescribed to dissolve the stones, but this often takes years and doesn't always work.

One of coconut oil's fatty acids is converted into monooctanoin in the body. Monooctanoin infused into the bile ducts of patients with gallstones showed complete gallstone dissolution in 50 to 75 percent of patients.[148] This is an effective and safe compound for eliminating the presence of gallstones in many patients, particularly those that are unable or unwilling to undergo surgical removal of the gallbladder. The infusion would have to be done by a medical professional in a health care setting.

HEALTH

61. HEAD LICE

WELL-BEING

Every year, it seems children are sent home from school with a note warning parents that there is an outbreak of head lice in the school. These tiny insects that infest human scalps are a source of panic and embarrassment, although having lice is not a sign of poor personal hygiene. They can fall off the head and land on carpet, bedding, towels, and stuffed animals, where they can lay their eggs and continue to grow for another day or two. Lice feed on the blood of the scalp and are readily transferred from one person to another through direct contact. A person may be infected for several weeks before itching begins. The itching is an allergic

BEAUTY

reaction to the louse saliva. The lice and nits (eggs) are difficult to see, but a close look around the ears and neckline may provide the best chance of glimpsing them. Over-the-counter and prescription medicated shampoos are used to kill the adult lice. The eggs are hard to get rid of, however, because they adhere to the hair shaft with a sticky substance that is difficult to wash out. A second treatment of medicated shampoo is recommended when the nits hatch.

Head lice are very common in school-age children worldwide. Current medications use one or a combination of insecticides to kill the lice. Because the lice are becoming resistant to a number of these commonly used treatments, a need for natural alternatives has arisen. In Israel, a study in school-aged children with active head lice infestations found that a spray containing coconut oil, anise oil, and ylang-ylang oil was 92.3 percent effective in getting rid of the lice compared to an insecticide, which yielded a 92.2 percent reduction in lice.[149] Another study found that using a coconut oil and anise oil spray was nearly twice as effective as the most commonly used medicated lice insecticide treatment, permethrin.[150] This significant difference in efficacy is likely due to the increasing resistance of lice to permethrin and underlines the importance of new and natural treatments for infestations. To remove lice, first rinse the hair with apple cider vinegar and allow the hair to dry. This loosens the glue that sticks the eggs to the hair shaft. Next, combine 1/4 cup melted coconut oil with 12 drops of anise oil and massage over the scalp and hair. Cover with a shower cap and leave it on overnight. In the morning, comb through the hair to remove dead eggs and lice. Shampoo as usual.

NUTRITION

HEALTH

WELL-BEING

BEAUTY

62. HEMORRHOIDS

Hemorrhoids are swollen veins in the rectum and anus. The walls of the veins can stretch and cause the blood vessels to bulge. Internal hemorrhoids are inside the rectum and can bleed into the stool. This area has few pain receptors, so hemorrhoids here generally do not hurt. External hemorrhoids are located on the anus where there are more pain-sensing nerves. These can be quite sore, especially during a bowel movement. They develop from a buildup of pressure in the lower rectum that can affect the flow of blood and cause the veins to swell. Straining during a bowel movement, pregnancy, or obesity can cause them. Hemorrhoids are extremely common and can explain bleeding, itching, pain, and inflammation. Topical creams or suppositories, cold packs, and oral pain relievers can help alleviate symptoms.

Reducing inflammation is key to shrinking hemorrhoids. Coconut oil has the anti-inflammatory compounds lauric acid and capric acid that can do this. They work by inhibiting specific protein complexes and enzymes that trigger the inflammatory process.[151] When swelling is reduced, the nerves in the area are no longer compressed and triggered to fire. Pain and itching subsides. Virgin coconut oil also contains polyphenols that act as anti-inflammatories and can aid the fatty acids in reducing symptoms. Apply coconut oil to a cotton ball and swab over the affected area. Do this several times a day, and in a few days, the swelling, pain, and itching should subside. Bowel movements will be easier and more comfortable.

63. HIGH CHOLESTEROL

Cholesterol is a waxy, fatlike substance found in cells. It is necessary for the body to make vitamin D, hormones, and bile acids that help digest food. We produce cholesterol on our own, but we also get it in saturated fat and cholesterol-laden foods. It comes in two forms: HDL (good) and LDL (bad). High cholesterol is when there are high levels of cholesterol in the blood, both HDL and LDL. When there is too much of LDL cholesterol in the body, however, it can build up in the arteries and increase the chances of getting coronary heart disease. Plaque containing cholesterol builds up inside the arteries and causes partial or full blockage, leading to narrowing and hardening of the arteries. This can lead to a heart attack or stroke. Statins are drugs commonly prescribed to lower LDL blood cholesterol. However, taking statins can cause intestinal problems and muscle inflammation.

Cholesterol levels respond well to changes in diet. Eating foods low in saturated fats and reducing intake of animal products, which are the primary contributors of cholesterol in the diet, will do wonders. Coconut oil, however, appears to be an exception to the rule as far as saturated fats are concerned. Because the fats are of medium chain length, they are absorbed directly into the bloodstream and carried to the liver, where they are distributed for energy. They do not contribute to elevating levels of LDL cholesterol in the body as most other saturated fats do. A study in women presenting with abdominal obesity found that adding coconut oil to the diet increased HDL cholesterol levels and had negligible effects on LDL cholesterol. Soybean oil, on the other hand, lowered

HDL and raised LDL levels, a very undesirable effect.[152] The rise in HDL cholesterol was confirmed by another study looking at the effects of coconut oil consumption on cholesterol levels in the body.[153] Having elevated levels of HDL cholesterol is important because they pick up LDL cholesterol and bring it to the liver. This reduces the levels of LDL cholesterol in the blood and decreases the risk of heart disease. As a preventative measure, consume 1 tablespoon of coconut oil a day. Try to substitute this for another type of saturated fat, such as butter, so total daily caloric intake will remain similar yet the nutrients from fat will have a much more beneficial effect on the cardiovascular system.

64. HORMONE LEVELS

Hormones are chemical messengers that travel throughout the body in the bloodstream and control most major bodily functions from mood and hunger to reproduction and growth. They are created by the endocrine glands: thyroid, parathyroid, thymus, pancreas, pituitary, hypothalamus, adrenal, pineal, ovaries, and testes. Each produces unique hormones with specific purposes, and all are needed for optimal physical, mental, and emotional health.

Saturated fats are essential building blocks for hormone production. Eating saturated fats has been associated with heart disease, but this is not the case with coconut oil. In fact, coconut oil, which is over 90 percent saturated fat, has been found to raise HDL (good) cholesterol levels without having an impact on LDL (bad) cholesterol levels.[154] This has a protective effect on the cardiovascular system. High amounts of HDL cholesterol also protect estrogen levels. This becomes particularly important for women as they approach menopause when estrogen levels tend to decline, bringing about physical and emotional changes. It is imperative that the body has adequate levels of saturated fats to produce hormones, and coconut oil can provide these without the detrimental effects other saturated fats are known to have.

65. IMMUNE SYSTEM

The immune system is the body's defense against bacteria, viruses, fungi, parasites, toxins, and allergens that can potentially invade the body and cause a lot of harm. Infants are more susceptible than adults because of their underdeveloped immune systems. A network of cells, tissues, and organs throughout the body work around the clock and communicate with each other. When a threat is detected, a defense is mounted. Because the immune system is so busy, any extra help through exogenous antimicrobial activity can prevent it from becoming overburdened. If this happens, disease can take over.

This is where coconut oil takes action. It has antifungal, antiviral, and antibacterial properties[155] which can attack any of these invading organisms and spare the immune system from getting involved. When consumed, medium-chain fatty acids in coconut oil and the derivatives formed from them in the body are able to destroy pathogenic cell membranes, interrupt the replicating process, and, ultimately, cause cell death. Massaging coconut oil onto the skin of preterm babies for their first twenty-eight days of life reduced their risk of bloodstream infections, increased daily weight gain, and improved skin condition over preterm infants in the control group who did not receive coconut oil on their skin.[156] This protective action of coconut oil shows promise as a very safe and effective preventative for infection in vulnerable newborns.

Phenolic acids, like those found in coconut oil, are also bioactive in a similar way to the fatty acids. They cross pathogen cell membranes, disrupt their metabolic functions, and cause their death. The phenolic acids are also antioxidants and are able to stop free radicals. Free radicals are responsible for damage to cells and tissues. They are unstable molecules actively looking for an electron. Free radicals attack the nearest stable molecule and steal one of their electrons, making that molecule a free radical. This begins a chain reaction, creating free radicals that can ultimately destroy the cell. The phenolic acids in coconut oil stabilize the free radicals by giving them one of their electrons. Damage is prevented so that the immune system doesn't have to clean up the aftereffects. Virgin coconut oil contains more antioxidants than refined oil[157] and is able to increase the activity of antioxidant enzymes in tissues, compared to other oils like sunflower and olive oil.[158]

Finally, taking coconut oil can help the liver, which is an integral part of the immune system. It is able to reduce fasting blood sugar levels in diabetic rats,[159] a job that usually falls to the liver. When blood sugar levels are too high, as often seen in diabetics, it's up to the liver to take in the excess sugar, which it stores or converts to fat. All the extra work can stress the liver and prevent it from working optimally. The entire immune system suffers. If the immune system doesn't seem to be healing wounds quickly or if multiple colds take hold over the season, it might need a little help. Take 1 tablespoon of coconut oil three times a day to boost the immune system.

66. Mosquito REPELLANT

Mosquitos are hardy pests that have been around for millions of years. They are tough to get rid of and even tougher to avoid when outside. The females bite humans in order to use their blood to develop their fertile eggs. As they do, they inject saliva into the skin, which can cause an immune system response. The results are tiny red spots in some people or itchy, swollen red welts in others. Mosquitos can smell their prey from up to fifty meters away and are attracted to carbon dioxide, movement, chemicals in sweat, and heat. Getting bitten by a mosquito may not seem like such a big deal, but these pesky insects can carry disease like West Nile virus, Zika virus, malaria, and yellow fever. To avoid getting bitten, many people use chemical repellant sprays or lotions on their skin. Chemical repellant paper strips worn on the body or placed in an outdoor area are used by some to avoid direct application of chemicals to the skin.

Many want to avoid chemical-based repellents and are turning to natural products as alternatives. One study tested a variety of herbal oils as mosquito repellents using coconut oil or mustard oil as the base. The commercial chemical repellent, dimethyl phthalate, was used as a control. Timur oil—from an indigenous plant in Nepal—in both coconut oil and mustard oil provided over six and a half hours of protection against mosquitos and was more effective than the commercial chemical repellent.[160] While it can be argued that it was the herb and not the carrier oil that provided the protection, the carrier oil is necessary to deliver the natural repellant safely to the skin. Next summer, try using coconut oil as a base and then adding to it timur, turmeric, neem, or other oils known to have insect-repelling activity.

NUTRITION

HEALTH

WELL-BEING

BEAUTY

67. MUSCLE GROWTH

As babies grow into children and then into adults, skeletal muscle tissue grows to keep up with the demands of the developing body. Many adults, however, choose to build muscle beyond the body's basic requirements in order to increase strength, endurance, or fat-burning muscle mass or to achieve a specific physique. Skeletal muscle is one of the most adaptable tissues in the human body and grows when the rate of muscle protein synthesis is faster than the rate of muscle protein breakdown.

One of the hormones involved in building muscle is insulin. Coconut oil stimulates the pancreas to secrete insulin,[161] which enters the bloodstream and travels to various tissues including muscle tissue. The cells of muscle tissue are lined with insulin receptors, and when insulin binds with them, the cells are able to take up glucose from the blood to use as energy. Along with glucose, amino acids and creatine enter the muscle cells. Insulin stimulates the cells to produce proteins from the incoming amino acids to be used in muscle growth and repair. It also increases blood flow to the muscles to deliver more nutrients, further enhancing the cell's muscle-building capabilities. Adding coconut oil to a smoothie (see Coconut Raspberry Smoothie on page 72) before a morning workout can help the body deliver the right nutrients to muscle cells to aid in recovery and growth.

68. NAIL FUNGUS

Fungal infections are extremely common and can infect any part of the body. When fungus targets the fingernails or toenails, white or yellow spots may begin to appear. These spots then merge to form patches and spread out. The nails become thicker, brittle, or discolored, and the edges start to crumble. The symptoms occur slowly and may eventually result in the nail detaching from the skin and falling off.

Fungal infections can actually be a sign of *Candida* overgrowth in the body. *Candida albicans* (*C. albicans*) is a very common fungus in humans and can grow out of control in people with weakened or compromised immune systems. The good bacteria in the gut cannot compete with *Candida,* and a systemic invasion may begin, which can show up as a fungal infection of the nails. Over-the-counter treatments are available, but they are not always effective and the chance of reoccurrence is high. Prescribed oral antifungal drugs can be used that allow new growth of the nail to be fungus free. This is a slow process and may cause a variety of side effects from a skin rash to liver disease. Medicated polishes and creams are also used, but these can take a year to get rid of the fungus. The nail can also be surgically removed, but it grows back slowly.

Coconut oil is an antifungal agent and can be used topically in the treatment of fungal infections. Four fatty acids found in coconut oil—caproic acid, caprylic acid, capric acid and lauric acid—were tested in a lab, and all four were able to inhibit *C. albicans* growth.[162] Another lab study found capric acid caused the fastest and most effective killing of three strains of *C. albicans*; lauric acid was the most active at lower concentrations, although it took longer.[163] Virgin coconut oil was found to be more effective than fluconazole, a common oral antifungal medication, when tested on various species of Candida.[164] Because some Candida species are becoming drug resistant, natural alternatives, like coconut oil, are readily available and accessible and can take their place. Before applying the oil, wash and completely dry the hand or foot. Add a small layer of oil over the affected areas and allow it to sink in. Reapply several times a day. Continue to do this daily until the nail grows out and is replaced by a healthy, fungus-free nail.

69. NEWBORN GROWTH

During the first month of life, newborns undergo astounding physical, emotional, and social developments. They tend to grow up to one and a half inches, add up to half a pound of weight, and learn to communicate. They begin to recognize faces and process sounds, smells, and tastes. To fuel these advancements, proper nutrition is key. Mother's milk contains all the nutrients, vitamins, and minerals in the correct amounts to help newborns grow and develop. Sometimes, though, breastfeeding is not an option, and infant formula can be used. These formulas also contain the right combination of nutrients, although they are missing some live cells and bioactive components that protect the newborn from infection and disease.

Research on well-term and preterm babies studied the growth effects of massage with either coconut oil, mineral oil, or placebo. Each baby was massaged four times a day from days two to thirty-one. In the preterm baby group, coconut oil significantly increased the rate of weight gain compared to mineral oil and placebo as well as the rate of length gain compared to placebo. In the well-term baby group, coconut oil significantly increased the rate of weight gain compared to placebo.[165] Massage with coconut oil can be used to increase newborn growth and is particularly effective in preterm babies.

Another way coconut oil can increase newborn growth is through additional caloric intake from mother's milk. Lauric acid and capric acid, both found in abundance in coconut oil, comprise about 20 percent of the saturated fats found in breast milk. Because the amount and variety of fatty acids found in breast milk are altered by the mother's diet, consuming coconut oil significantly increases the amounts of these fatty acids in breast milk within six hours. These amounts remain elevated for up to twenty-four hours.[166] When the newborn breastfeeds, the mother passes these compounds on to her baby, who is easily able to digest them due to the fatty acids' relatively small size. Fat molecules have more than twice the calories as other nutrients and can aid in newborn weight gain.

70. NUTRIENT ABSORPTION

Food provides the nutrients to the body necessary for growth, maintenance, and survival. Eating a diet rich in vitamins and minerals, complex carbohydrates, and good fats should provide the basic ingredients for a healthy, thriving individual. Sometimes,

NUTRITION

HEALTH

WELL-BEING

BEAUTY

however, all this good food cannot be used to its full potential because the body is not able to completely digest and absorb the nutrients. Microbial infection, inflammation, and an overgrowth of bad intestinal bacteria are a few factors that can affect nutrient absorption.

Coconut oil is made up mostly of antimicrobial medium-chain fatty acids that can destroy certain bacterial, viral, fungal, and parasitic infections by disrupting their plasma membranes, leaking cytoplasmic contents, interrupting replication, and/or preventing maturation. Removing the source of the infection allows the intestinal tissues to heal and restore absorptive capability. The medium-chain fatty acids are thought to reduce intestinal inflammation and improve the absorption of the fat-soluble vitamins A, D, E, and K as well as vitamin B12.[167] Recent studies have found that when either a long-chain fatty acid formula or a 50/50 medium- to long-chain fatty acid formula were supplemented to patients, the absorption rate of vitamin E doubled with the 50/50 formula. This is likely due to the action of the medium-chain fatty acids.[168] Coconut oil was also shown to enhance the uptake of carotenoids from tomatoes when fed to gerbils.[169] Finally, coconut oil can decrease the bad bacteria in the gut that can overtake the good bacteria. The good bacteria assist in the metabolism of nutrients and help with the absorption of certain compounds through the intestinal wall.

71. PINK EYE

Conjunctivitis, or pink eye, is an infection of the clear tissue over the white part of the eye and the lining of the eyelid. When the blood vessels in the whites of the eye become inflamed, they are more visible, and the result is a reddish or pink-looking eye. The eyes may burn, itch, blur, and tear. They often produce a yellow discharge that crusts over the eyelashes and prevents the eye from opening after sleep. The infection can affect one eye or both and is commonly caused by bacteria, viruses, allergens, or irritants. Bacterial and viral pink eye are contagious, so it's important to keep hands away from the eyes to prevent the spread of the infection. Antibiotics are prescribed for bacterial infections, but viral ones have to run their course. Both types tend to resolve within a week. Pink eye caused by allergens or irritants can clear when the source of infection has been identified and removed.

A home remedy for pink eye is coconut oil. Make sure it is unprocessed and pure so no unwanted chemicals are present. Coconut oil has antibacterial and antiviral properties and can help eliminate the source of infection by destroying the membranes of these microbes and causing their death. Lauric acid and capric acids are also anti-inflammatories[170] and can reduce swelling of the blood vessels and lessen eye redness, itching, and burning. The eye should feel soothed soon after application. It may seem daunting to put anything in or around the eye, but virgin coconut oil has been proven to be as safe as saline or commercial eye drops.[171] Melt the coconut oil and apply a generous amount to a cotton ball. Once cooled to a pleasing temperature, wipe around the eye, squeezing the cotton ball gently to allow some oil to enter the whites of the eyes. Blink several times to distribute the oil over the eye and under the eyelid. Throw away the cotton ball after a single use to prevent reinfection.

72. PROTECTS LIVER

The liver is the largest internal organ in the body. It filters toxins out of the bloodstream to prevent them from damaging tissues. When the liver tissue itself becomes damaged, it has the ability to regenerate and make new, healthy tissue. When the damage gets too extensive, however, liver disease sets in and the liver no longer functions as it should. A number of conditions can cause liver disease, including hepatitis A, B, and C, cirrhosis of the liver, nonalcoholic fatty liver disease, and alcoholic hepatitis. Symptoms include abdominal swelling and pain, bruising, fatigue, loss of appetite, and jaundice.

A study published using laboratory rats showed that pretreatment with 10 milliliters/kilogram of virgin coconut oil significantly reduced liver damage when 3 grams/kilogram of acetaminophen was administered to the rats to induce liver damage. The control group saw increased liver weights, inflammation, and necrosis.[172] Coconut oil was also shown to protect the liver in rats against the toxic effects of trimethoprim-sulfamethoxazole, a broad-spectrum antibiotic.[173]

Nonalcoholic fatty liver disease is becoming more prevalent today with the rise in diabetes, but coconut oil provides a protective effect by targeting the factors that contribute to this condition. It reduces oxidative stress on the liver by providing stable saturated fatty acids rather than easily-oxidized mono- and polyunsaturated fatty acids. It decreases blood glucose and increases insulin secretion[174] to aid the liver in regulating blood glucose levels and reducing inflammation.[175] The antioxidant ability of the polyphenols in coconut oil can also guard against alcohol-induced liver damage. Coconut oil has the potential to be used as a natural supplement for the prevention and treatment of liver disease.

73. PSORIASIS

Psoriasis is a common skin condition caused when skin cells grow ten times faster than normal. This overabundance of cells creates raised red plaques with silvery scales on the surface of the skin. These patches can be itchy and painful, and the skin can dry out, crack, and bleed. Nails can also become pitted and discolored. Up to 30 percent of people with psoriasis also have psoriatic arthritis and experience pain and swelling in their joints. Most cases of psoriasis go through periods of flare-up and remission and can be triggered by stress, certain medications, infection, skin injury, smoking, or cold weather. These triggers send a faulty immune system into action. Some of the body's white blood cells attack healthy skin cells, provoking other immune responses that cause the proliferation of skin cells, redness, inflammation, and other symptoms. There is no cure, but psoriasis can be managed with topical treatments, light therapy, and oral or injectable drugs.

To date, the best that can be hoped for in those with psoriasis is to keep the condition in remission as long as possible and to treat

NUTRITION

HEALTH

WELL-BEING

BEAUTY

the symptoms of flare-up as they occur. Coconut oil boosts the immune system by providing chemicals that work on processes in the body that are normally the responsibility of the immune system. This relieves stress on the system so it doesn't become overburdened and depressed. Coconut oil has polyphenols that act as antioxidants and clean up free radical damage. If psoriatic arthritis has developed, the polyphenols can stop the action of reactive oxygen species and free radicals that cause joint degradation in arthritis.[176] When polyphenols from virgin coconut oil were used to treat arthritic rats, swelling was greatly reduced after three weeks of treatment.[177]

Coconut oil also has antifungal, antiviral, and antibacterial properties,[178, 179] which can destroy invading organisms. In fact, *Candida* is one of the triggers of psoriasis that worsens the condition and makes it last longer. The quantity of *Candida* is significantly higher in patients with psoriasis compared to healthy adults.[180] Coconut oil is highly effective at destroying *Candida*,[181] with capric acid and lauric acid showing the most activity against the yeast. Swelling and pain are attenuated.

Applying coconut oil directly onto the affected area several times a day should moisturize the skin and reduce itching and swelling. Consuming up to 3 tablespoons a day in divided doses during an active flare-up will help provide support to the immune system and could destroy any invading pathogenic triggers.

74. SINUSITIS

The hollow air spaces within the bones around the nose are the sinuses. When they become swollen and inflamed, sinusitis develops. The tissues produce thick yellow or green mucus, which drains into the nose or down the back of the throat. Breathing through the nose becomes difficult, and there may be pain, pressure, or tenderness around the eyes or nose that worsens when bending over. Sometimes, the pain extends to the ears, jaws, and teeth. Acute sinusitis begins as a cold and usually resolves itself within ten days. Chronic sinusitis lasts for at least twelve weeks and may be caused by allergies, respiratory tract infections, diseases, or nasal problems. Corticosteroids or antibiotics are sometimes given to reduce inflammation and destroy the infection, if bacterial.

Lauric acid and capric acid, constituents in coconut oil, have been shown to reduce swelling, in part, by inhibiting specific protein complexes and enzymes that trigger inflammation.[182] This allows tissue in the airways to shrink, mucus to be removed, and the flow of air through the sinuses to be greatly increased. The medium-chain fatty acids and the phenolic acids are all antimicrobial compounds and can prevent the spread of infection to others. At the onset of a cold, add a tablespoon of coconut oil to soup or to your morning cup of coffee. Do this several times a day to drain away mucus, reduce inflamed tissue, and open the airways for easier breathing. Applying coconut oil to either side of the nose has been reported to work for some, while others prefer to apply coconut oil directly in their sinuses. To do that, add a tablespoon of melted oil to warm saline water in a neti pot and pour through the sinuses. Alternatively, add a few milliliters of melted oil from a dropper into the nasal passages. If trying this method, be sure the oil is not too hot.

....

75. SLOW METABOLISM

Chemical reactions in the body convert everything consumed into nutrients used to maintain good health and proper functioning of cells in the entire body. Some of these reactions break down compounds to be used as energy. Other reactions build compounds that the cells use to carry out their jobs and to grow and repair tissues. In some people, these reactions proceed at a slower pace than in others. There are many reasons for a slow metabolism. With age, muscle mass declines and fat accounts for more body weight. Muscle burns more energy than fat. Women generally have higher percentages of fat in their bodies than men, so metabolism tends to be slower in women. People on diets may restrict their calories too much, causing a slowing down in metabolism to conserve energy. Some conditions, like an underactive thyroid or diabetes, are also associated with slow metabolisms, while certain medications and genetics play a role as well.

The medium-chain fatty acids in coconut oil play a role in boosting metabolism. They fuel reactions in the body that are necessary to drive processes forward to create substances needed in various parts of the body for functioning. Without adequate fuel, the reactions would be slow or stop altogether, causing a sluggish metabolism, which impacts overall health. Coconut oil does not act like most of the other fats consumed in our diets. The relatively small size of the medium-chain fatty acids, which constitute about 90 percent of the oil, allows them to be absorbed directly from the intestine without having to be broken down like other larger fatty acids. They go directly to the liver rather than being stored in fat cells and then can be used by the body to fuel metabolic processes. They are easily digested and a quick source of energy, which is why they are added to nutritional drinks for athletes and to infant formulas. To enhance flavor and satiety without increasing the waistline, try substituting coconut oil for any of the commonly used vegetable oils like olive, canola, or sunflower oil.

76. SORE THROAT

A sore throat is pain, irritation, and itchiness of the throat that worsens upon swallowing. The glands of the neck might be swollen, the voice may be hoarse, and small, white patches can even appear on the tonsils. The main culprits are viral and bacterial infections, but smoke, dry air, and allergies can cause a sore throat too. When the tissues lining the throat become irritated or infected, blood rushes to the area and brings with it germ-fighting cells. The blood vessels in the tissues swell, putting pressure on the nerve endings and causing pain. Sore throats from viral infections usually last five to seven days and are treated with over-the-counter pain relievers. Bacterial infections, like strep throat, require antibiotics.

Coconut oil can be used to treat the symptoms and the cause of a sore throat. It has the ability to inhibit specific protein complexes and enzymes that trigger inflammation[183] and has been shown to reduce swelling and pain.[184] This will make swallowing much less painful. Coconut oil is also a strong topical remedy to rid the body of infections and can effectively attack both bacterial and viral sources. Taking coconut oil will decrease the duration of infection by allowing its antibacterial and antiviral acids to attack the pathogens by disrupting their membranes and causing cell death. If the infection is severe and antibiotics are required, coconut oil can still be used as a complement to bring extra fighting power. Melt a tablespoon of virgin coconut oil in the mouth and gargle several times a day.

77. STEATORRHEA

Stools that have excess fat in them are termed steatorrhea. It happens when the body is unable to absorb fats, resulting in light-colored, soft, bulky, and foul-smelling stools. They may float or stick to the sides of the toilet. Abdominal pain and cramping often accompany this condition. The loss of excessive fat by excretion usually means inadequate levels have been absorbed and are available to the body. This becomes particularly important in patients needing calories for growth or those that have difficulty maintaining a healthy weight. Steatorrhea usually results from disease or intestinal infections. The absorption of fat is dependent on bile, which the liver produces and stores in the gallbladder. It is also dependent on the quantity and quality of digestive enzymes and the intestinal function, which is influenced by inflammation or intestinal resection surgery.

Coconut oil consists mainly of medium-chain fatty acids and can be absorbed directly through the intestinal wall without being digested in the intestines like most other fats and oils that are made up of long-chain fatty acids. If a lack of digestive enzymes is the issue, coconut oil bypasses that problem. Good-quality bile is needed to break down fats in the digestive tract. If the bile is thick and sticky, it doesn't emulsify the fats and they cannot be absorbed and used by the body. Coconut oil does not need bile for digestion and absorption. While it cannot cure steatorrhea, the ability of coconut oil to be absorbed and used by the body despite factors present preventing most other fats from doing so allows it to be used in cases of steatorrhea to maintain weight, decrease offensive stools, improve abdominal discomfort, and enhance nutrition.[185]

78. STREP THROAT

Strep throat is a common bacterial infection of the throat and tonsils. The symptoms come on very suddenly and cause a sore, red, inflamed throat with white patches or tiny red spots on the back of the roof of the mouth. It is often accompanied by a fever, tender lymph nodes, and headache. *Streptococcus pyogenes*, or group A streptococcus, is the bacteria responsible for this contagious infection. It is spread when a healthy person inhales contaminated air droplets from the cough or sneeze of an infected person. It can also be acquired from sharing food or drinks. Even touching contaminated surfaces can pick up the bacteria and cause illness if the bacteria are then transferred to the mouth, nose, or eyes. Once transmitted, it takes two to five days for symptoms to develop. As long as symptoms are present, the infection is contagious. Oral antibiotics are prescribed to shorten the duration of the illness,

NUTRITION

HEALTH

WELL-BEING

BEAUTY

reduce the risk of spreading the infection to other parts of the body, and prevent the spread of the bacteria to others.

Lauric acid constitutes approximately 50 percent of coconut oil. It has antibacterial activity and, when ingested, is partially converted into monolaurin. Monolaurin is even more biologically active than lauric acid. It has been shown to be effective at inactivating group A streptococci, the bacteria responsible for strep throat. It dissolves the fats in the envelope surrounding the bacteria, causing the membrane to disintegrate.[186] Monolaurin also interferes with the communication between the bacteria and host cells and prevents the bacteria from gaining entrance into the cells to replicate.[187] Additionally, coconut oil has anti-inflammatory properties that can reduce swelling and pain while it works to destroy the strep bacteria. Try gargling several times a day with a solution of 1/2 cup of warm water, a pinch of salt, and 1 tablespoon of melted coconut oil. This should soothe the area and reduce swelling.

79. SWIMMER'S EAR

Water that remains in the ear after swimming can cause an infection inside the outer ear canal. The warm, moist environment is the perfect breeding ground for bacteria that are commonly found in water. They will readily invade the skin and multiply. The infection causes itching and redness that can escalate to severe pain in and around the ear, discharge of pus, fever, and partial or complete blockage of the ear canal. To stop the infection, doctors commonly prescribe antibiotics and eardrops that contain both antibiotics and steroids. Taking over-the-counter pain medications such as ibuprofen is also recommended.

Coconut oil has the ability to destroy the bacteria causing the infection and help relieve the symptoms of swimmer's ear. It contains anti-inflammatory compounds, lauric and capric acids, which have the ability to inhibit specific protein complexes and enzymes that trigger inflammation.[188] This reduces swelling and redness and allows the tissues to relieve pressure on the nerves to reduce pain. Coconut oil's antibacterial agents can destroy the source of the infection so the ear tissues can regain their health. The medium-chain fatty acids in coconut oil are able to disrupt bacterial membranes and cause cell death. Lay on one side with the affected ear facing up. Fill the ear canal with melted coconut oil—roughly 1/4 of a teaspoon—and let it remain there for twenty minutes. Turn the head to the side and drain the liquid. Continue this each day until the infection clears up. If the eardrum is perforated or if treating a child with ear tubes, do not use this method.

80. THRUSH

When the yeast *C. albicans* overgrows in the lining of the mouth, white lesions develop on the tongue and inner cheeks and may cause redness and soreness. This is called thrush. While *Candida* are normally present in the body, their numbers are kept in check by the immune system. Sometimes, when the immune system is weakened by disease or drugs, *Candida* grows out of control and causes an infection. It is most common in babies and the elderly, but it is also seen in adults with compromised immune systems. This condition is not generally serious, but if left unchecked, the yeast can spread to other areas of the body, like the lungs, heart, liver, and digestive tract. Most cases are controlled with antifungal medications.

Coconut oil is highly effective at destroying *Candida*.[189] In a laboratory setting, four fatty acids found in coconut oil— lauric, capric, caproic, and caprylic—were tested against *C. albicans*. All inhibited growth of the yeast. Capric acid was then assessed for its ability to inhibit the growth of *Candida* in the mouths of rodents. After three applications, yeast numbers were found to be significantly decreased.[190] Another study showed capric acid and lauric acid were the most active against the yeast. These acids were able to disintegrate the plasma membranes of the yeast and destroy the cells.[191] Virgin coconut oil was even found to be more effective than fluconazole, a common oral antifungal medication, when tested on various species of *Candida*.[192] For children, melt a teaspoon of coconut oil by adding the oil to a small bowl and placing it in a larger bowl filled with an inch of hot (not boiling) water. Once melted, swish the coconut oil around the mouth for five minutes. Spit out into the trash. Repeat several times a day. Adults can use 1/2 to 1 tablespoon of oil in the same way. If a baby has thrush, clean a pacifier and rub a layer of coconut oil over the nipple. Allow the baby to suckle the pacifier.

81. TOOTH DECAY

The mouth is full of bacteria. Some are helpful, and others are harmful. The harmful bacteria form a sticky, colorless substance that adheres to the teeth and gum line. This is called plaque. Plaque loves to feed on sugars and starches, so nearly every meal provides plaque with fuel for growth. As the bacteria in the plaque feed on the sugars, they produce acids. These acids demineralize the tooth surface by extracting calcium and phosphate from the enamel. Saliva tries to neutralize the acids and provide the missing minerals so the tooth enamel can remineralize. When demineralization happens faster than remineralization, the tooth begins to decay, creating holes or cavities. Cavities are a major oral health concern and affect up to 90 percent of schoolchildren and the majority of adults. The only treatment for cavities is to drill out the decay and fill the hole with composite resins, porcelain, or amalgams.

Once a cavity has begun, the process cannot be reversed. The best course of action is to prevent tooth decay before it starts. A good oral hygiene routine is essential and should involve flossing and brushing twice daily. Reducing sugar consumption can also help to lower acid output from bacteria that cause enamel erosion. As an added measure, coconut oil can be used to inhibit bacterial growth in the mouth. Lauric acid in coconut oil can decrease plaque formation and prevent hydroxyapatite, an essential strengthening ingredient in teeth, from dissolving.[193] Coconut oil was also found to be as effective as an antimicrobial oral rinse in reducing *Streptococcus mutans*, the most common organism causing dental cavities.[194] After brushing in the morning, swish coconut oil around the mouth for several minutes and spit out into the trash. This should help reduce cavity-inducing bacterial counts and protect the teeth from acid erosion.

NUTRITION

HEALTH

WELL-BEING

BEAUTY

82. WARTS

Warts are small skin growths caused by the human papillomavirus (HPV). They are usually flesh-colored and contain small black dots, which are actually clotted blood vessels. The hands and the fingers are the most common areas where they are found, which is not surprising since the virus is contagious. If warts occur on the soles of the feet, they are called plantar warts. Most warts go away on their own, but it may take a year or two. Many people find them embarrassing and opt to get rid of them using salicylic acid medications, freezing, or laser treatments. These can cause pain, blistering, and scarring.

Coconut oil can be used to remove common and plantar warts. The medium-chain fatty acids in the oil penetrate the skin and have antiviral properties that are thought to destroy HPV after several weeks of application. If the wart is small and soft, massage warmed coconut oil directly over the area several times a day. If the wart is large and tougher, file the skin over the wart to expose the tender layers underneath. Rub the warmed coconut oil over the area. Alternatively, soak a cotton ball in warm coconut oil and press over the wart. Secure the cotton ball with a bandage. After several weeks, the wart should shrink and the tissue should heal.[195]

83. WEIGHT LOSS

When the body accumulates too much body fat, it increases the risk of health problems like diabetes, heart disease, and certain cancers. Losing weight can improve or prevent any weight-induced conditions. Fat accumulates on the body when more calories are eaten than burned. The body stores these excess calories as fat. Exercising and eating a healthy diet with appropriate calorie intake will help burn the stored fat and reduce body weight.

Consuming virgin coconut oil has been found to safely reduce waist circumference in obese men over a four-week period.[196] This result was independently confirmed in women presenting with abdominal obesity.[197] Dietary medium-chain fatty acids are thought to aid in weight loss by increasing the number of fat cells broken down and used for energy. This effect was observed in rat cells pretreated with caprylic acid, one of coconut oil's medium chain fatty acids.[198]

During the weight-loss process, people often report reaching plateaus where they no longer seem to be able to continue losing weight, despite continued efforts with exercise and dieting. This is because metabolism slows down as weight is lost. Coconut oil can amp up metabolism by providing an easily digested source of energy. The medium-chain fatty acids, which make up most of the oil, are absorbed directly into the bloodstream, go to the liver, and become available to the cells as fuel. The medium-chain fatty acids in coconut oil can also increase thermogenesis—heat production in the body. The more heat the body produces, the more calories it burns. This is needed for weight loss. Ingesting between five grams and ten grams of medium-chain fatty acids significantly increases thermogenesis in the body compared to consuming long-chain fatty acids.[199]

Finally, coconut oil increases nutrient absorption.[200, 201] Amino acids, fats, sugars, starches, vitamins, and minerals are essential to metabolic processes, and without these key nutrients, metabolism slows down. Adding coconut oil to meals can increase the breakdown of fat cells, burn more calories, and increase metabolism, all of which will aid in losing weight.

84. WOUND HEALING

Wounding the skin is a very common occurrence and happens to everyone. Whether it's slicing the tip of the finger while dicing carrots or slipping on gravel and scraping a knee, cuts and scrapes tear the skin tissue and often cause bleeding. If the wound is deep, bleeds heavily, or has an object embedded in it, seek medical attention. If it's minor, however, it can be addressed at home. Wash your hands with soap and water. Clean the cut or scrape by pouring cool, clean water over it to remove dirt and debris. Then wash with soap and water. Once clean, an antibiotic ointment can be applied.

This is where coconut oil comes in handy. A study on the effects of virgin coconut oil on wound healing in rats found that coconut oil mended wounds much faster than the control group that received no coconut oil. Skin tissue formed over the wound more quickly, collagen cross-linking was increased, and more new blood vessels formed.[202] Coconut oil is also an antibacterial agent and can attack and kill bacteria that find their way into an open wound. This discourages infection and helps the immune system heal the skin. Sometimes, there is pain and swelling in and around the cut. Coconut oil can reduce these symptoms by inhibiting specific protein complexes and enzymes that trigger inflammation.[203] Coconut oil can be applied directly to the skin and consumed every day to support the body during the wound healing process.

85. XEROSIS

Dry skin is common, and everyone experiences it at one time or another. When skin gets extremely dry, however, it can feel tight and itchy and look flaky, scaly, and cracked. This is called xerosis. It is most common during the winter months or in low humidity environments. The skin cells lose water and oils. These need to be replenished to return the skin to its normal smooth, healthy appearance. Regular use of oil-based moisturizers is recommended.

Coconut oil has been used as a moisturizer for centuries, but until recently, the efficacy and safety had not been thoroughly investigated. Using coconut oil as a natural therapeutic moisturizer would provide a cost-effective and widely available treatment for xerosis. Fortunately, coconut oil was found to be as safe and effective as mineral oil when used in patients with mild to moderate xerosis. After two weeks of use, coconut oil significantly improved skin hydration and increased lipid levels on the skin surface.[204] While mineral oil sits on the surface of the skin, coconut oil can penetrate the layers and moisturize deeper within as well as provide antimicrobial activity against any pathogens that may find their way through dry, cracked skin. It's safe, effective, and protective.

CHAPTER 4

MANAGING BEAUTY

OVERHAUL YOUR LOOK

86. ACNE

Acne is a skin condition that results in pimples, blackheads, whiteheads, cysts, nodules, and papules. It often appears on the face, but it can also show up on the neck, chest, back, upper arms, shoulders, and buttocks. Acne is the most common skin problem in the United States. It happens when dead skin cells stick together with sebum (oil) inside the pore. They become trapped. Bacteria living on the skin can sometimes get stuck in the pores with the dead skin cells. This provides a perfect breeding ground for them, and they quickly multiply. The skin then becomes inflamed. If the acne goes deeper into the skin, a nodule or cyst forms. Typically, acne appears in teenagers and young adults, but it can affect anyone, even babies. Scars and dark spots on the skin can result. Mild acne can be treated with over-the-counter products that contain benzoyl peroxide or salicylic acid. It takes four to eight weeks of using the product for acne to clear. For best resolution, a dermatologist should treat more severe cases. Prescription grade topical treatments, whole body treatments like antibiotics, or office procedures involving lasers, lights, or chemicals may be used.

Lauric acid in coconut oil has strong antibacterial properties. A study tested whether lauric acid was effective against

Propionibacterium acnes (*P. acnes*)—bacteria living in the follicles and pores of skin. They can grow in numbers and trigger inflammation, resulting in acne. Lauric acid was able to inhibit bacterial growth at levels much lower than the commonly used topical medication benzoyl peroxide. Human sebocytes—which protect the skin from drying out—were unaffected by lauric acid.[205] Applying coconut oil to acne after washing the face—rather than other medicated topical products like benzoyl peroxide—can clear the skin by destroying the bacteria that clog the pores with debris. This helps reduce swelling, redness, and pain associated with large, rounded blemishes. They become less noticeable and bothersome to the individual.

If acne is severe and antibiotics are prescribed, coconut oil may be supplemented alongside them to provide extra bacteria-fighting power. Consuming coconut oil supports a healthy digestive system, which is especially important through a course of antibiotics, which destroy the good bacteria in the gut. And the digestive system must be working properly to absorb all the nutrients needed for glowing skin.

87. AGING SKIN

The process of getting older involves many changes in the body. Arteries stiffen, bones lose density, memory declines, skin thins, and wrinkles appear. The rate at which these processes take place varies from person to person. Genetics and illness play a role in when and how we age, but our diet and lifestyle significantly impact the process. There are many theories of aging, but the free radical theory is growing in popularity as an explanation. It is

NUTRITION

HEALTH

WELL-BEING

BEAUTY

thought that free radicals are responsible for age-related damage of cells and tissues. Free radicals are unstable molecules actively looking for an electron. They attack the nearest stable molecule and steal one of their electrons, making that molecule a free radical as well. This begins a chain reaction of creating free radicals that ultimately can destroy the cell.

The key to stopping these free radicals lies in the presence of antioxidants. Coconut oil contains medium-chain fatty acids, which increase antioxidant activity,[206] and polyphenols, potent antioxidant compounds themselves. These compounds sidle up to free radicals and give them an electron. Now they are happy and leave neighboring molecules alone. Cells and tissues continue to live, and the aging process is slowed. This happens throughout the body, from the liver to the skin. Virgin coconut oils have higher antioxidant levels than refined coconut oils[207], so when applying coconut oil to the skin, use virgin oil.

Coconut oil promotes the formation of skin tissue and increases collagen cross-linking. [208] Collagen gives bodies support and structure. It is a main component of skin, hair, and nails, and as collagen is lost, the signs of aging set in. Consuming coconut oil orally or applying it topically will slow aging and give a healthier and more youthful appearance. As a note of caution, coconut oil is comedogenic and can clog pores and cause acne in individuals with oily skin or those prone to breakouts. Experiment with amounts of oil and application.

88. DAMAGED HAIR

There are about one hundred thousand to one hundred and fifty thousand hairs on the human head. Each strand of hair consists of three layers, with the outer layer, or cuticle, protecting the inner two layers. When the hair is healthy, the scales of the cuticle overlap tightly and protect the inner layers. When it becomes damaged, however, the scales of the cuticle loosen and separate, exposing the layers underneath. The hair looks dry and dull and may break easily. Now the inner layers can become damaged from exposure to the UV rays of the sun, heat, pollution, chlorine, or any of the array of chemicals found in hair products and treatments.

A common ingredient found in many hair products is coconut oil, and with good reason. The fatty acids in coconut oil are attracted to proteins in the hair shaft, prompting the oil to bind with them. This prevents protein loss and maintains hair strength and structure. When coconut oil was used either before or after washing, it was shown to reduce protein loss in both damaged and undamaged hair.[209] In addition to protein loss, hair can be damaged from the constant swelling and contracting of the hair shaft as it goes from wet to dry. This causes the hair to stretch and break. Coconut oil maintains hair strength by limiting the swelling of hair when wet.[210] Gently melt a few tablespoons of coconut oil in a bowl. Massage into wet hair, beginning at the bottom and working toward the scalp. Wrap the hair in a shower cap and let sit for about thirty minutes. Then shampoo as normal. The hair should feel smooth, silky, and nourished.

NUTRITION

HEALTH

WELL-BEING

BEAUTY

89. DENTURES

Gum disease, tooth decay, or injury can all damage teeth to the point where they fall out or need to be removed. Dentures can replace missing teeth and improve facial appearance and the ability to eat and speak. Complete dentures replace all the teeth in the mouth, and partial dentures replace only the teeth that are missing. Dentures should be removed at night and cleaned with a soft bristle toothbrush to remove food, plaque, bacteria, and yeast. They should be stored in water overnight to prevent the dentures from drying out and warping.

If dentures are not cleaned properly, they can cause irritation of the gums and bad breath. Brushing dentures does remove food and plaque, but it is not very effective in removing bacteria and yeasts. If a disinfecting agent is not used in addition to brushing, the denture wearer runs the risk of infection of the mucosal membranes. This is often caused by *Candida* species, commonly found in the mouth. If left alone, they multiply and thrive on the gums underneath the dentures. This causes a condition known as denture-induced stomatitis, which is an inflammation and redness of the gums. Coconut oil is highly effective at destroying *Candida*,[211] with capric acid and lauric acid showing the most activity against the yeast. The acids were able to disintegrate the plasma membranes of the yeast and destroy the cells.[212] Virgin coconut oil was even found to be more effective than fluconazole, a common oral antifungal medication, when tested on various species of *Candida*.[213] A study in denture wearers found that cleansing dentures with coconut soap made from coconut oil and then soaking in a solution of 0.05 percent bleach was effective at reducing stomatitis.[214] This should be done nightly to help keep microbial numbers low. Coconut soap can be purchased online, at some farmer's markets, and in health stores.

90. EARWAX REMOVAL

Earwax is the yellowish-brown substance produced in the ears that is made up of dead skin cells, hair, sebum, and sweat. The body produces earwax to lubricate and protect the inner ears from infection or irritation caused by germs, dust, and water. However, too much wax can cause hearing loss or an overgrowth of bacteria leading to infection. Ears are designed to be self-cleaning. Fine hairs in the outer ear canal sweep the wax to the outer ear where it dries, flakes, and falls out. Often, people use cotton swabs to try to remove earwax, but this pushes most of the wax deeper into the ear canal. Over time, the wax gets compacted near the ear canal and can affect hearing or produce earaches or infections. In these cases, ears must be cleaned.

An effective at-home treatment is to use warmed coconut oil. Gently melt a teaspoon of oil in a bowl placed in warm water. Fill an ear dropper with the oil. Lie on one side with the impacted ear facing up. Add three to four drops of coconut oil into the ear. Cover the ear with a cotton ball. Wait fifteen minutes. Sit up and tilt the ear down. The coconut oil lubricates the ear canal and softens the wax, allowing it to flow out of the ear. The fatty acids in the oil are antimicrobial and can improve infections by destroying pathogens trying to make a home in the canal. This is also a wonderful method for regular ear cleaning. For excessive amounts of impacted earwax, several applications of coconut oil will be needed.

91. TEETH WHITENER

Bright, white teeth make for a beautiful smile and give a younger and healthier appearance. There are many products in stores that claim to whiten teeth. Whitening toothpastes remove surface stains with mild abrasive agents and can achieve about one shade of difference. Whitening gels, strips, and trays contain hydrogen peroxide or other bleaching agents, which lighten deep within the tooth. Results usually last about four months. Some mouthwashes contain ingredients to whiten teeth, but they are less effective, and results are often not seen for twelve weeks. Dentists can also dramatically whiten teeth in their offices in one visit. Tooth sensitivity and tissue irritation are a few side effects of the bleaching process.

Bacteria in the mouth build up a biofilm on the teeth called plaque. Plaque can cause the teeth to become discolored and look yellow. However, coconut oil contains lauric acid that is antibacterial and can decrease plaque formation.[215] It is as effective as an antimicrobial oral rinse in reducing *Streptococcus mutans*, a common organism in dental biofilms.[216] A study in teenage children performing coconut oil pulling every day for thirty days found significant reductions in plaque.[217] Coconut oil is clearly effective in eliminating the bacteria in the mouth responsible for yellowing of the teeth.

According to *Reader's Digest*, up to 78 percent of people experience tooth sensitivity when whitening with products that use forms of peroxide. Coconut oil is a gentle alternative to whiten teeth without sensitivity, allowing for daily use and no pain. Each morning, put 1 to 2 teaspoons of coconut oil into the mouth and allow it to melt. Swish around the mouth for about twenty minutes. Spit into the trash can. Rinse with warm water and brush the teeth.

OVERHAUL YOUR COSMETICS

92. DEODORANT

Sweating is a natural function of the body used to reduce body heat. Sweat itself is odorless. The warm, moist environment, however, is a breeding ground for bacteria, and they thrive in the armpit in these conditions. The bacteria break down keratin protein on the surface of the skin and produce odor-causing fatty acids and ammonia. To reduce armpit odor, wash regularly and keep the armpit dry. Most people use antiperspirants to reduce sweating or deodorants to mask odor.

Because sweating is a natural process to regulate body temperature and remove toxins from the body, allowing the body to sweat is recommended. Deodorants can help mask odor for a period of time, but bacteria can overpower even the most pungent scents.

The best way to be odor-free is to make sure the bacteria don't have a chance to grow in the armpits. Coconut oil has antibacterial medium-chain fatty acids that can destroy bacteria and keep away any offending odors. Simply take a small amount of hardened coconut oil onto the fingertips and massage into the armpits. Add a drop of essential oil like lavender, peppermint, or bergamot to boost the aroma and antibacterial power of the deodorant.

93. EYE MAKEUP REMOVER

Many women and some men use makeup around the eyes to draw attention, define, and accentuate the beauty of the eyes and brows. Eyeliner, eye shadow, brow pencils, concealer, foundation, and mascara are commonly used to achieve this. At the end of the day before going to bed, it is essential that eye makeup is removed so that bacteria cannot grow and potentially harm the eye tissue. Removing makeup also prevents it from dirtying pillowcases and bedsheets. Wipes and solutions to remove eye makeup must be non-irritating and formulated to easily wipe off all traces of product. Still, many of these makeup removal products contain sodium lauryl sulfate, poloxamer 184, triethanolamine, colorants, and fragrance, among other ingredients that can be irritating to sensitive skin or have contaminants that can cause any number of reactions.

Coconut oil is nourishing to the eye and non-irritating. In fact, it can be used directly in the eye to aid in clearing microbial infections and has been proven to be as safe as saline or commercial eye drops.[218] Coconut oil contains no irritants but, instead, hydrating

NUTRITION

fatty acids that break up the makeup and allow it to be readily lifted from the skin and lashes. The only downside is that if some oil gets into the eyes, then vision can blur for a few minutes, but that goes away quickly. It is not harmful and can actually benefit the eye by destroying any rogue bacteria that have landed there from makeup residue. Apply some coconut oil to the fingertips and massage over the eye area. Take a dry cotton ball or cotton pad and gently wipe the coconut oil and makeup off. You'll be amazed at how easy and effective it is!

HEALTH

94. FRAGRANCE

Some people have an affinity for sweet smells, others for flowery scents, while still others prefer strong musky or woodsy aromas. Fortunately, there is no shortage of pleasing fragrances to suit every taste and mood. They are added to a huge array of products, from cosmetics and cleaners to garbage bags and tissues. When "fragrance" or "perfume" is listed as an ingredient on a product, it more often than not is a combination of aromatic chemicals. The US Department of Health and Human Services reports there are over 5000 different fragrance chemicals used in products. Using products with synthetic chemicals may cause dermatitis, disrupt hormones, or even be toxic to the brain. Make sure to read the ingredients and stay away from synthetic fragrances.

WELL-BEING

Finding products that use coconut oil as their fragrance will provide the benefits of a wonderfully aromatic product without the harmful side effects of synthetic fragrances. There are over 600 cosmetic products using coconut oil as an ingredient, so shampoos,

BEAUTY

lotions, scrubs, and masks that have coconut oil as their fragrance are readily available. Or, instead of buying products, try using your coconut oil alone as a body moisturizer for a fresh beachy smell or as a carrier oil for any number of blended essential oils to create a customized and unique perfume or musk. Add sugar into the mix, and you have a marvelous facial exfoliator. There are abundant possibilities to create fragrant homemade cosmetic products with coconut oil that can save money, nourish the skin, and take the place of harmful chemical fragrances.

95. LEAVE-IN HAIR CONDITIONER AND DETANGLER

Maintaining long, sleek tresses or thick, bouncy curls without the constant struggle of detangling knots may seem impossible. Tangled hair can lead to breakage. When the hair is healthy, the scales of the cuticle overlap tightly and protect the inner layers. When the hair shaft breaks, the scales of the cuticle separate, exposing the layers underneath. The hair looks wispy, frizzy, dry, and dull. Hair that isn't properly conditioned will tangle much more easily than if it is infused with moisture. Conditioners smooth the scales of the hair down and create a seal so the hair is easier to brush and preserve in a tangle-free state.

Coconut oil is able to penetrate the hair shaft because of its low molecular weight and straight chain.[219] It infuses its nourishing oil to the inside of the hair shaft, smooths the cuticles, and locks in moisture. Hair is strengthened by the fatty acids in coconut oil binding to the proteins in the hair shaft, preventing their loss. The oil also counters damage by limiting the swelling of the hair when wet.[220] Over time, constant swelling and contracting injures the hair so that it breaks more easily. The end result of applying coconut oil is hair that is healthy, moisturized, and sleek. After shampooing and towel blotting wet hair, add a dime-size amount of melted coconut oil into the palm. Rub hands together and begin to work the oil into the hair. Brush easily and effortlessly with a wide-tooth comb. It may take some adjustment with the amount of oil to determine the optimal amount needed for your hair length, but the result should be hair that is perfectly moisturized and tangle-free without feeling or looking greasy.

96. MAKEUP BRUSH CLEANER

Makeup brushes come in a variety of sizes and shapes, and each are tailored for specific applications. Powder, contour, blush, eyeshadow, mascara, and lipstick brushes are just some of the different kinds used on the face, eyes, and lips. The handles are typically wooden or plastic, while the bristles can be either synthetic or natural. Synthetic bristles are easier to clean because the synthetic filaments don't tend to trap or absorb pigments. Natural bristles are made out of real animal hair, so they can become damaged and break. They are also porous like the hairs on our head. The porosity allows natural brushes to absorb products and pigments, which can breed bacteria if not cleaned on a regular basis.

Using brushes with weeks' worth of old makeup bound to the bristles can spread bacteria and irritate the skin and eyes. Not only can these bacteria clog pores and cause acne, but they can also infect the eyes, causing inflammation, tenderness, and redness. Coconut oil can be used to clean makeup brushes by loosening product from the bristles so that it can be rinsed away. Massage coconut oil into the bristles for a few minutes and rinse thoroughly with warm water. All product should easily wash away. Next, massage oil once again into the bristles and let the brush sit for half an hour to allow the antibacterial properties of the medium-chain fatty acids to destroy any remaining bacteria. Rinse once more with warm water and blot on a paper towel.

97. MOISTURIZER

Having toned and moisturized skin gives the appearance of youth. Smooth, even texture without blemishes, dark spots, acne scars, or blotches is the hallmark of beauty, and having beautiful skin like this is something everyone desires. Living a healthy lifestyle, eating properly, and getting exercise and plenty of sleep will help achieve this. Aging, however, causes the skin to begin to sag and wrinkles to form. Skin looks dull and tired. Oftentimes, more help is needed.

Coconut oil has been used as a moisturizer for centuries. Topical application of coconut oil was tested for its moisturizing properties in patients with very dry skin. It was able to increase the measureable amount of surface lipids and improved skin hydration. Patch test results also determined coconut oil is safe.[221] Coconut oil stimulates collagen cross-linking,[222] which can improve skin firmness and elasticity. This reduces sagging skin and the look of fine lines and wrinkles. The result is smoother, younger-looking skin. The antioxidants in coconut oil also prevent free radicals from UV rays and toxins from damaging skin cells. Apply the oil directly to the body to improve the look and feel of the skin.

While coconut oil can freely be used on the body, caution is advised when using on the face. This oil has a high comedogenic rating and is more likely to clog pores and cause acne breakouts in susceptible people.

98. PERSONAL LUBRICANT

Personal lubricants are used to reduce friction or dryness during intercourse. They are water, oil, or silicone based, and they often contain a number of chemicals that are questionable for vaginal health. The following have all been found in personal lubricants: chlorhexidine, propylene glycol, and phenoxyethanol (all of which can irritate the delicate skin in the vagina); parabens that can mimic estrogens and may be linked to an increased risk of breast cancer; and glycerin, a sugar alcohol that can encourage an overgrowth of *Candida* in the vagina, leading to a yeast infection. Other constituents can have impurities in them that can lead to a number of other health issues.

Opt for coconut oil as a lubricant for its safety, efficacy, and wonderful aroma. Coconut oil coats the skin to reduce chafing and readily penetrates the skin due to its small molecular size and weight, making it a great moisturizer. The introduction of foreign bacteria or yeast from a partner will fall prey to the action of coconut oil's antimicrobial compounds, and the potential growth and spread of a vaginal infection will be prevented. Lauric and capric acids in coconut oil can kill *Candida* species and numerous bacteria by destroying their cell membranes.[223, 224] One note of caution is to avoid using coconut oil (or any oil) as a lubricant if latex or polyisoprene condoms are used. The oil can weaken the condom. If the oil has stained clothes or sheets, sprinkle them with baking soda before washing and the oil should come right out.

99. SOAP

Soap has been around for thousands of years and was made by mixing fats, oils, and salts. The first soaps were not made for washing the body but instead were created to clean goods and textiles or to use medicinally in the treatment of skin diseases. It wasn't until the 19th century that bars of soap were used for personal hygiene. Commercial soaps available in every grocery store, supermarket, big box store, and pharmacy often contain parabens, phthalates, artificial colors, and synthetic fragrances. Some of these are linked to cancer, irritate the skin, or cause hormonal issues.

We are becoming more aware that the foods we eat have tremendous impact on our health. Just as important are the products we put on our skin. Our skin provides a protective barrier to the inside of our body, but many chemicals found in the products we apply topically are able to penetrate the skin. They enter the bloodstream and are carried throughout the body, where they can have any number of adverse effects. Replacing chemical-laden soap with a natural alternative, like coconut oil soap, will hydrate the skin with beneficial fatty acids and provide antimicrobial protection to ward off infection and disease. Numerous recipes for coconut oil soap are available online and can be made at home using only coconut oil, lye, water, and essential oil (optional). Other recipes call for additional ingredients, mostly other oils. Many vegetable oils go rancid after a relatively short period of time if not kept in a cool, dark, dry place. Coconut oil, however, is very shelf stable, so it is ideal to use in soap and will remain good for up to a year.

100. SUNSCREEN

Excessive exposure to the sun can cause sunburn, promote the development of wrinkles and sagging skin, and increase the risk of melanoma or squamous cell carcinoma. It is important to receive some sun so that the skin can make vitamin D, which is essential for bone growth and remodeling, immune function, and neuromuscular activity. Just as important, however, is to protect the skin from the harmful ultraviolet rays of the sun. Suncreens do just this. They come as lotions, sprays, gels, and sticks and are applied topically. They either absorb the ultraviolet rays or reflect sunlight. Many suncreens block only ultraviolet B sunlight, which causes sunburns. But it is ultraviolet A sunlight that increases skin damage and the risk of skin cancers. Broad-spectrum suncreens will block both types of rays. Some of the ingredients used in commercially available suncreens include

PABA, phenylbenzimidazole sulfonic acid, sulisobenzone, and octocrylene (among many others) that can irritate the skin, increase damaging reactive oxygen species, and cause DNA defects.

Coconut oil is a natural sunscreen that has SPF (sun protection factor) of 7.[225] This means that 1/7th of the sun's ultraviolet B radiation reaches the skin. It blocks only ultraviolet B rays, meaning it will help prevent the skin from burning, but it doesn't provide protection against ultraviolet A rays, which increase the risk of cancer and photodermatitis. Coconut oil makes an ideal natural, safe, and moisturizing sunscreen when spending small amounts of time in the sun. If extended periods are to be spent outdoors, reapply frequently and consider supplementing with a product that supplies ultraviolet A protection as well.

101. MOUTHWASH

Using mouthwash as part of an oral hygiene regimen is optional, but many choose to include it. Most mouthwashes are antiseptic and are used to decrease the microbes in the mouth to prevent cavities, gingivitis, and bad breath. Others are advertised as reducing inflammation, pain, or dry mouth caused by infection or disease. About 20 milliliters of mouthwash is gargled for thirty seconds or more then spit out into the sink.

If bad breath is a problem, using coconut oil as a mouthwash can remove the bacteria from the mouth and stop their metabolic byproducts from emitting offensive odors. The medium-chain fatty acids in the oil have antibacterial properties that disrupt the bacterial cell membranes, resulting in cell death. It can also be used to eliminate much of the *Candida* yeast in the mouth to prevent localized and systemic infections that can spread to other areas of the body. Virgin coconut oil was even found to be more effective than fluconazole, a common oral antifungal medication, when tested on various species of *Candida*.[226]

For those taking mouthwash to reduce inflammation of the gums, lauric and capric acids in coconut oil are able to reduce tissue swelling, which can also alleviate pain. The alcohol content in some mouthwashes can dry the tissue in the mouth, but coconut oil is moisturizing and can penetrate the outer layers of the skin. It has been found to be hydrating and increase lipid levels on the tissue surface.[227] To use as a mouthwash, combine a teaspoon of coconut oil with half a teaspoon of baking soda and two drops of peppermint essential oil. Swish around the mouth for thirty seconds and spit into the toilet or garbage.

NUTRITION

HEALTH

WELL-BEING

BEAUTY

NOTES

1. Marina, A. M., Y. B. Che Man, and I. Amin. 2009. "Virgin coconut oil: emerging functional food oil." *Trends in Food Science & Technology* 20 (10): 481–7.
2. Srivastava, Y., A. D. Semwal, and M. S. L. Swamy. 2013. "Hypocholesterimic effects of cold and hot extracted virgin coconut oil (VCO) in comparison to commercial coconut oil: evidence from a male wistar albino rat model." *Food Science and Biotechnology* 22 (6): 1501–8.
3. Brito, N. M., S. Navickiene, L. Polese, E. F. Jardim, R. B. Abakerli, and M. L. Ribeiro. 2002. "Determination of pesticide residues in coconut water by liquid-liquid extraction and gas chromatography with electron-capture plus thermionic specific detection and solid-phase extraction and high-performance liquid chromatography with ultraviolet detection." *Journal of Chromatography A* 957 (2): 201–9.
4. Fries, J. H., and M. W. Fries. 1983. "Coconut: a review of its uses as they relate to the allergic individual." *Annals of Allergy, Asthma & Immunology* 51 (4): 472–81.
5. Online Natural Medicines website, https://naturalmedicines.therapeuticresearch.com.
6. Wang, Jianhong, Xiaoxiao Wang, Juntao Li, Yiqiang Chen, Wenjun Yang, and Liying Zhang. 2015. "Effects of dietary coconut oil as a medium-chain fatty acid source on performance, carcass composition and serum lipids in male broilers." *Asian-Australasian Journal of Animal Sciences* 28 (2): 223–30.
7. Assunção, M. L., H. S. Ferreira, A. F. dos Santos, C. R. Cabral Jr., and T. M. Florêncio. 2009. "Effects of dietary coconut oil on the biochemical and anthropometric profiles of women presenting abdominal obesity." *Lipids* 44 (7): 593–601.
8. Page, Kathleen A., Anne Williamson, Namyi Yu, Ewan C. McNay, James Dzuira, Rory J. McCrimmon, and Robert S. Sherwin. 2009. "Medium-chain fatty acids improve cognitive function in intensively treated type 1 diabetic patients and support in vitro synaptic transmission during acute hypoglycemia." *Diabetes* 58 (5): 1237–44.
9. Institute for Quality and Efficiency in Health Care (IQWiG). 2013. "High cholesterol: Does reducing the amount of fat in your diet help?" *Informed Health Online*: 1–4.

10. Wang, "Effects of dietary coconut oil as a medium-chain fatty acid source on performance, carcass composition and serum lipids in male broilers."

11. Assunção, "Effects of dietary coconut oil on the biochemical and anthropometric profiles of women presenting abdominal obesity."

12. Feranil, A. B., P. L. Duazo, C. W. Kuzawa, and L. S. Adair. 2011. "Coconut oil is associated with a beneficial lipid profile in pre-menopausal women in the Philippines." *Asia Pacific Journal of Clinical Nutrition* 20 (2): 190–5.

13. Nafar, F., and K. M. Mearow. 2014. "Coconut oil attenuates the effects of amyloid-β on cortical neurons in vitro." *Journal of Alzheimer's Disease* 39 (2): 233–7.

14. Henderson, S. T., J. L. Vogel, L. J. Barr, F. Garvin, J. J. Jones, and L. C. Costantini. 2009. "Study of the ketogenic agent AC-1202 in mild to moderate Alzheimer's disease: a randomized, double-blind, placebo-controlled, multicenter trial." *Nutrition and Metabolism (London)* 6: 31.

15. Newport, M. T., T. B. VanItallie, Y. Kashiwaya, M. T. King, and R. L. Veech. 2015. "A new way to produce hyperketonemia: use of ketone ester in a case of Alzheimer's disease." *Alzheimer's & Dementia* 11 (1): 99–103.

16. Arthritis Foundation. "Arthritis Facts." http://www.arthritis.org/about-arthritis/understanding-arthritis/arthritis-statistics-facts.php.

17. Wruck, C. J., A. Fragoulis, A. Gurzynski, L. O. Brandenburg, Y. W. Kan, K. Chan, J. Hassenpflug, S. Freitag-Wolf, D. Varoga, S. Lippross, and T. Pufe. 2011. "Role of oxidative stress in rheumatoid arthritis: insights from the Nrf2-knockout mice." *Annals of the Rheumatic Diseases* 70 (5): 844–50.

18. Vysakh, A., M. Ratheesh, T. P. Rajmohanan, C. Pramod, S. Premlal, B. Girish Kumar, and P. I. Sibi. 2014. "Polyphenolics isolated from virgin coconut oil inhibits adjuvant induced arthritis in rats through antioxidant and anti-inflammatory action." *International Immunopharmacology* 20 (1): 124–30.

19. Marina, A. M., Y. B. Che Man, S. A. H. Nazimah, and I. Amin. 2009. "Chemical properties of virgin coconut oil." *Journal of the American Oil Chemists' Society* 86 (4): 301–7.

20. Aly, Mona M., Maisa A. Shalaby, Samar S. Attia, Shaimaa H. El Sayed, Soheir S. Mahmoud. 2013. "Therapeutic effect of lauric acid, a medium chain saturated fatty acid, on Giardia lamblia in experimentally infected hamsters." *Parasitologists United Journal* 6 (1): 89–98.

21. Law, K. S., N. Azman, E. A. Omar, M. Y. Musa, N. M. Yusoff, S. A. Sulaiman, and N. H. Hussain. 2014. "The effects of virgin coconut oil (VCO) as supplementation on quality of life (QOL) among breast cancer patients." *Lipids in Health and Disease* 13: 139.

22. Narayanan, A., S. A. Baskaran, M. A. Amalaradjou, and K. Venkitanarayanan. 2015. "Anticarcinogenic properties of medium chain fatty acids on human

colorectal, skin and breast cancer cells in vitro." *International Journal of Molecular Sciences* 16 (3): 5014–27.

23. Projan, S. J., S. Brown-Skrobot, P. M. Schlievert, F. Vandenesch, and R. P. Novick. 1994. "Glycerol monolaurate inhibits the production of beta-lactamase, toxic shock toxin-1, and other staphylococcal exoproteins by interfering with signal transduction." *Journal of Bacteriology* 176 (14): 4204–9.

24. Altekruse, Sean F., Norman J. Stern, Patricia I. Fields, and David L. Swerdlow. 1999. "Campylobacter jejuni—An Emerging Foodborne Pathogen." *Emerging Infectious Diseases* 5 (1): 28–35.

25. Thormar, H., H. Hilmarsson, and G. Bergsson. 2016. "Stable concentrated emulsions of the 1-monoglyceride of capric acid (monocaprin) with microbicidal activities against the food-borne bacteria Campylobacter jejuni, Salmonella spp., and Escherichia coli." *Applied and Environmental Microbiology* 72 (1): 522–6.

26. National Center for HIV/AIDS, Viral Hepatitis, STD, and TB Prevention. Division of STD Prevention. 2016. "Sexually Transmitted Disease Surveillance 2015." Centers for Disease Control and Prevention. https://www.cdc.gov/std/stats15/std-surveillance-2015-print.pdf.

27. Farley, T. A., D. A. Cohen, and W. Elkins. 2003. "Asymptomatic sexually transmitted diseases: the case for screening." *Preventive Medicine* 36 (4): 502–9.

28. Korenromp, E. L., M. K. Sudaryo, S. J. de Vlas, R. H. Gray, N. K. Sewankambo, D. Serwadda, M. J. Wawer, and J. D. Habbema. 2002. "What proportion of episodes of gonorrhoea and chlamydia becomes symptomatic?" *International Journal of STD & AIDS* 13 (2): 91–101.

29. Rours, G. I. J. G., L. Duijts, H. A. Moll, L. R. Arends, R. de Groot, V. W. Jaddoe, A. Hofman, E. A. P. Steegers, J. P. Mackenbach, A. Ott, H. F. M. Willemse, E. A. E. van der Zwaan, R. P. Verkooijen, and H. A. Verbrugh. 2011. "Chlamydia trachomatis infection during pregnancy associated with preterm delivery: a population-based prospective cohort study." *European Journal of Epidemiology* 26 (6): 493–502.

30. Bergsson, G., J. Arnfinnsson, S. M. Karlsson, O. Steingrímsson, and H. Thormar. 1998. "In vitro inactivation of Chlamydia trachomatis by fatty acids and monoglycerides." *Antimicrobial Agents and Chemotherapy* 42 (9): 2290–4.

31. Nishino, H., M. Murakoshi, X. Y. Mou, S. Wada, M. Masuda, Y. Ohsaka, Y. Satomi, and K. Jinno. 2005. "Cancer prevention by phytochemicals." *Oncology* 69 (Suppl. 1): 38–40.

32. Burton, A. F. 1991. "Oncolytic effects of fatty acids in mice and rats." *The American Journal of Clinical Nutrition* 53 (Suppl. 4): 1082S–1086S.

33. Mañé, Josep, Elisabet Pedrosa, Violeta Lorén, Isabel Ojanguren, Lourdes Fluvià, Eduard Cabré, Gerhard Rogler, and Miquel A. Gassull. 2009. "Partial replacement of dietary (n-6) fatty acids with medium-chain triglycerides decreases the incidence of spontaneous colitis in interleukin-10-deficient mice." *Journal of Nutrition* 139 (3): 603–10.

34. Iranloye, Bolanle, Gabriel Oludare, and Makinde Olubiyi. 2013. "Anti-diabetic and antioxidant effects of virgin coconut oil in alloxan induced diabetic male Sprague Dawley rats." *Journal of Diabetes Mellitus* 3 (4): 221–6.

35. Page, "Medium-chain fatty acids improve cognitive function in intensively treated type 1 diabetic patients and support in vitro synaptic transmission during acute hypoglycemia."

36. Neal, Elizabeth G., Hannah Chaffe, Ruby H. Schwartz, Margaret S. Lawson, Nicole Edwards, Geogianna Fitzsimmons, Andrea Whitney, and J. Helen Cross. 2008. "The ketogenic diet for the treatment of childhood epilepsy: a randomised controlled trial." *The Lancet Neurology* 7 (6): 500–6.

37. Khoramnia, Anahita, Afshin Ebrahimpour, Raheleh Ghanbari, Zahra Ajdari, and Oi-Ming Lai. 2013. "Improvement of medium chain fatty acid content and antimicrobial activity of coconut oil via solid-state fermentation using a Malaysian *Geotrichum candidum.*" *BioMed Research International* 2013: 954542.

38. DebMandal, Manisha, and Shyamapada Mandal. 2011. "Coconut (Cocos nucifera L.: Arecaceae): in health promotion and disease prevention." *Asian Pacific Journal of Tropical Medicine* 4 (3): 241–7.

39. Thormar, "Stable concentrated emulsions of the 1-monoglyceride of capric acid (monocaprin) with microbicidal activities against the food-borne bacteria Campylobacter jejuni, Salmonella spp., and Escherichia coli."

40. Intahphuak, S., P. Khonsung, and A. Panthong. 2010. "Anti-inflammatory, analgesic, and antipyretic activities of virgin coconut oil." *Pharmaceutical Biology* 48 (2): 151–7.

41. Bergsson, G., O. Steingrímsson, and H. Thormar. 2002. "Bactericidal effects of fatty acids and monoglycerides on Helicobacter pylori." *International Journal of Antimicrobial Agents* 20 (4): 258–62.

42. Sun, C. Q., C. J. O'Connor, and A. M. Roberton. 2003. "Antibacterial action of fatty acids and monoglycerides against Helicobacter pylori." *FEMS Immunology and Medical Microbiology* 36 (1–2): 9–17.

43. Peedikayil, Faizal C., Prathima Sreenivasan, and Arun Narayanan. 2015. "Effect of coconut oil in plaque related gingivitis—a preliminary report." *Nigerian Medical Journal* 56 (2): 143–7.

44. Bergsson, G., O. Steingrímsson, and H. Thormar. 1999. "In vitro susceptibilities of Neisseria gonorrhoeae to fatty acids and monoglycerides." *Antimicrobial Agents and Chemotherapy* 43 (11): 2790–2.

45. Lieberman, S., M. G. Enig, and H. G. Preuss. 2006. "A review of monolaurin and lauric acid natural virucidal and bactericidal agents." *Alternative & Complementary Therapies* 12 (6): 310–14.

46. DebMandal, "Coconut (Cocos nucifera L.: Arecaceae): In health promotion and disease prevention."

47. Projan, "Glycerol monolaurate inhibits the production of beta-lactamase, toxic shock toxin-1, and other staphylococcal exoproteins by interfering with signal transduction."

48. Yano, Masahiko, Masanori Ikeda, Ken-ichi Abe, Hiromichi Dansako, Shogo Ohkoshi, Yutaka Aoyagi, and Nobuyuki Kato. 2007. "Comprehensive analysis of the effects of ordinary nutrients on hepatitis C virus RNA replication in cell culture." *Antimicrobial Agents and Chemotherapy* 51 (6): 2016–27.

49. Thormar, H., G. Bergsson, E. Gunnarsson, G. Georgsson, M. Witvrouw, O. Steingrímsson, E. de Clercq, and T. Kristmundsdóttir. 1999. "Hydrogels containing monocaprin have potent microbicidal activities against sexually transmitted viruses and bacteria in vitro." *Sexually Transmitted Infections* 75 (3): 181–5.

50. Lieberman, "A review of monolaurin and lauric acid natural virucidal and bactericidal agents."

51. Dayrit, C. S. 2000. "Coconut oil in health and disease: Its and monolaurin's potential as cure for HIV/AIDS." *Pharmacology University of the Philippines*: 1–14.

52. Enig, M. G. 1997. "Coconut oil: An anti-bacterial, anti-viral ingredient for food, nutrition and health." AVOC Lauric Symposium. Manila, Philippines.

53. Ross, R., and L. Harker. 1976. "Hyperlipidemia and atherosclerosis." *Science* 193 (4258): 1094–1100.

54. Feranil, "Coconut oil is associated with a beneficial lipid profile in pre-menopausal women in the Philippines."

55. Henry, G. E., R. A. Momin, M. G. Nair, and D. L. Dewitt. 2002. "Antioxidant and cyclooxygenase activities of fatty acids found in food." *Journal of Agricultural and Food Chemistry* 50 (8): 2231–4.

56. Assunção, "Effects of dietary coconut oil on the biochemical and anthropometric profiles of women presenting abdominal obesity."

57. Alves, Naiane Ferraz Bandeira, Suênia Porpino, Matheus Monteiro, Thyago Queiroz, Karen Montenegro, and Valdir Braga. 2014. "Coconut oil supplementation reduces blood pressure and oxidative stress in spontaneously hypertensive rats." *BioMed Central Proceedings* 8 (Suppl. 4): 68.

58. Mendis, S., R. W. Wissler, R. T. Bridenstine, and F. J. Podbielski. 1989. "The effects of replacing coconut oil with corn oil on human serum lipid profiles and platelet derived factors active in atherogenesis." *Nutrition Reports International* 40 (4): 773–82.

59. DebMandal, "Coconut (Cocos nucifera L.: Arecaceae): In health promotion and disease prevention."

60. Gold, S. 1971. "Use of Parawax with coconut oil in the treatment of lipodystrophy." *Canadian Medical Association Journal* 105 (4): 346.

61. Dawson, P. L., G. D. Carl, J. C. Acton, and I. Y. Han. 2002. "Effect of lauric acid and nisin-impregnated soy-based films on the growth of Listeria monocytogenes on turkey bologna." *Poultry Science* 81 (5): 721–6.

62. Zakaria, Z. A., M. S. Rofiee, M. N. Somchit, A. Zuraini, M. R. Sulaiman, L. K. Teh, M. Z. Salleh, and K. Long. 2011. "Hepatoprotective activity of dried- and fermented-processed virgin coconut oil." *Evidence-Based Complementary and Alternative Medicine* 2011: 142739.

63. Marina, A. M., Y. B. Man, S. A. Nazimah, and I. Amin. 2009. "Antioxidant capacity and phenolic acids of virgin coconut oil." *International Journal of Food Sciences and Nutrition* 60 (Suppl. 2): 114–23.

64. Nevin, K. G., and T. Rajamohan. 2006. "Virgin coconut oil supplemented diet increases the antioxidant status in rats." *Food Chemistry* 99 (2): 260–6.

65. Zakaria, "Hepatoprotective activity of dried- and fermented-processed virgin coconut oil."

66. Marina, "Antioxidant capacity and phenolic acids of virgin coconut oil."

67. Nevin, "Virgin coconut oil supplemented diet increases the antioxidant status in rats."

68. "Malaria." 2017. Centers for Disease Control and Prevention. https://www.cdc.gov/malaria/.

69. Al-Adhroey, A. H., Z. M. Nor, H. M. Al-Mekhlafi, A. A. Amran, and R. Mahmud. 2011. "Evaluation of the use of Cocos nucifera as antimalarial remedy in Malaysian folk medicine." *Journal of Ethnopharmacology* 134 (3): 988–91.

70. Arora, R., R. Chawla, R. Marwah, P. Arora, R. K. Sharma, V. Kaushik, R. Goel, A. Kaur, M. Silambarasan, R. P. Tripathi, and J. R. Bhardwaj. 2011. "Potential of complementary and alternative medicine in preventive management of novel H1N1 flu (swine flu) pandemic: thwarting potential disasters in the bud." *Evidence-Based Complementary and Alternative Medicine* 2011: 586506.

71. Projan, "Glycerol monolaurate inhibits the production of beta-lactamase, toxic shock toxin-1, and other staphylococcal exoproteins by interfering with signal transduction."

72. Feranil, "Coconut oil is associated with a beneficial lipid profile in pre-menopausal women in the Philippines."

73. Assunção, "Effects of dietary coconut oil on the biochemical and anthropometric profiles of women presenting abdominal obesity."

74. Alves, "Coconut oil supplementation reduces blood pressure and oxidative stress in spontaneously hypertensive rats."

75. Mendis, "The effects of replacing coconut oil with corn oil on human serum lipid profiles and platelet derived factors active in atherogenesis."

76. Liau, Kai Ming, Yeong Yeh Lee, Chee Keong Chen, and Aida Hanum G. Rasool. 2011. "An open-label pilot study to assess the efficacy and safety of virgin coconut oil in reducing visceral adiposity." *ISRN Pharmacology* 2011: 949686.

77. Assunção, "Effects of dietary coconut oil on the biochemical and anthropometric profiles of women presenting abdominal obesity."

78. Iranloye, "Anti-diabetic and antioxidant effects of virgin coconut oil in alloxan induced diabetic male Sprague Dawley rats."

79. Gorres, K. L., D. Daigle, S. Mohanram, and G. Miller. 2014. "Activation and repression of Epstein-Barr Virus and Kaposi's sarcoma-associated herpesvirus lytic cycles by short- and medium-chain fatty acids." *Journal of Virology* 88 (14): 8028–44.

80. Galli, F., M. Piroddi, C. Annetti, C. Aisa, E. Floridi, and A. Floridi. 2005. "Oxidative stress and reactive oxygen species." *Contributions to Nephrology* 149: 240–260.

81. Alves, "Coconut oil supplementation reduces blood pressure and oxidative stress in spontaneously hypertensive rats."

82. Iranloye, "Anti-diabetic and antioxidant effects of virgin coconut oil in alloxan induced diabetic male Sprague Dawley rats."

83. Bai, X. C., D. Lu, J. Bai, H. Zheng, Z. Y. Ke, X. M. Li, and S. Q. Luo. 2004. "Oxidative stress inhibits osteoblastic differentiation of bone cells by ERK and NF-κB." *Biochemical and Biophysical Research Communications* 314 (1): 197–207.

84. Abujazia, Mouna Abdelrahman, Norliza Muhammad, Ahmad Nazrun Shuid, and Ima Nirwana Soelaiman. 2012. "The effects of virgin coconut oil on bone oxidative status in ovariectomised rat." *Evidence-Based Complementary and Alternative Medicine* 2012: 525079.

85. Hayatullina, Zil, Norliza Muhammad, Norazlina Mohamed, and Ima-Nirwana Soelaiman. 2012. "Virgin coconut oil supplementation prevents bone loss in osteoporosis rat model." *Evidence-Based Complementary and Alternative Medicine* 2012: 237236.

86. Shea, J. C., M. D. Bishop, E. M. Parker, A. Gelrud, and S. D. Freedman. 2003. "An enteral therapy containing medium-chain triglycerides and hydrolyzed peptides reduces postprandial pain associated with chronic pancreatitis." *Pancreatology* 3 (1): 36–40.

87. Ogbolu, D. O., A. A. Oni, O. A. Daini, and A. P. Oloko. 2007. "In vitro anti-microbial properties of coconut oil on Candida species in Ibadan, Nigeria." *Journal of Medicinal Food* 10 (2): 384–7.

88. Lieberman, "A review of monolaurin and lauric acid natural virucidal and bactericidal agents."

89. Biasi-Garbin, Renata Perugini, Fernanda de Oliveira Demitto, Renata Claro Ribeiro do Amaral, Magda Rhayanny Assunção Ferreira, Luiz Alberto Lira Soares, Terezinha Inez Estivalet Svidzinski, Lilian Cristiane Baeza, and Sueli Fumie Yamada-Ogatta. 2016. "Antifungal potential of plant species from Brazilian caatinga against dermatophytes." *Revista do Instituto de Medicina Tropical de Sao Paulo* 58: 18.

90. Johny, A. K., S. A. Baskaran, A. S. Charles, M. A. Amalaradjou, M. J. Darre, M. I. Khan, T. A. Hoagland, D. T. Schreiber, A. M. Donoghue, D. J. Donoghue, and K. Venkitanarayanan. 2009. "Prophylactic supplementation of caprylic acid in feed reduces Salmonella Enteritidis colonization in commercial broiler chicks." *Journal of Food Protection* 72 (4): 722–7.

91. Van Immerseel, F., J. de Buck, F. Boyen, L. Bohez, F. Pasmans, J. Volf, M. Sevcik, I. Rychlik, F. Haesebrouck, and R. Ducatelle. 2004. "Medium-chain fatty acids decrease colonization and invasion through hilA suppression shortly after infection of chickens with Salmonella enterica serovar Enteritidis." *Applied and Environmental Microbiology* 70 (6): 3582–7.

92. Thormar, "Stable concentrated emulsions of the 1-monoglyceride of capric acid (monocaprin) with microbicidal activities against the food-borne bacteria Campylobacter jejuni, Salmonella spp., and Escherichia coli."

93. Narayanan, "Anticarcinogenic properties of medium chain fatty acids on human colorectal, skin and breast cancer cells in vitro."

94. Fife, Bruce. 2005. *Coconut Cures: Preventing and Treating Common Health Problems with Coconut.* Colorado Springs, Colorado: Piccadilly Books, Ltd.

95. Khoramnia, "Improvement of medium chain fatty acid content and antimicrobial activity of coconut oil via solid-state fermentation using a Malaysian *Geotrichum candidum.*"

96. Rouse, Mark S., Margalida Rotger, Kerryl E. Piper, James M. Steckelberg, Matthew Scholz, Jeffrey Andrews, and Robin Patel. 2005. "In vitro and in vivo evaluations of the activities of lauric acid monoester formulations against Staphylococcus aureus." *Antimicrobial Agents and Chemotherapy* 49 (8): 3187–91.

97. Kasai, M., N. Nosaka, H. Maki, Y. Suzuki, H. Takeuchi, T. Aoyama, A. Ohra, Y. Harada, M. Okazaki, and K. Kondo. 2002. "Comparison of diet-induced thermogenesis of foods containing medium- versus long-chain triacylglycerols." *Journal of Nutritional Science and Vitaminology (Tokyo)* 48 (6): 536–40.

98. "Trichomoniasis: CDC Fact Sheet." 2017. Centers for Disease Control and Prevention. https://www.cdc.gov/std/trichomonas/stdfact-trichomoniasis.htm.

99. DebMandal, "Coconut (Cocos nucifera L.: Arecaceae): In health promotion and disease prevention."

100. El-Sherbini, G. M., K. M. Ibrahim, E. T. El-Sherbini, N. M. Abdel-Hady, and T. A. Morsy. 2010. "Efficacy of Punica granatum extract on in-vitro and in-vivo control of Trichomonas vaginalis." *Journal of the Egyptian Society of Parasitology* 40 (1): 229–44.

101. Bergsson, "Bactericidal effects of fatty acids and monoglycerides on Helicobacter pylori."

102. Sun, "Antibacterial action of fatty acids and monoglycerides against Helicobacter pylori."

103. Selvarajah, Malarvili, Zuraini Ahmad, Zainul Amiruddin Zakaria, Hoe Siong Chiong, Yoke Kin Yong, Kamariah Long, and Muhammad Nazrul Hakim. 2015. "Comparative investigation into the anti-ulcer activity of virgin coconut oil and coconut oil in pylorus ligated animal model." *TANG* 5 (4): 28.

104. Khoramnia, "Improvement of medium chain fatty acid content and antimicrobial activity of coconut oil via solid-state fermentation using a Malaysian *Geotrichum candidum*."

105. DebMandal, "Coconut (Cocos nucifera L.: Arecaceae): In health promotion and disease prevention."

106. Thormar, "Stable concentrated emulsions of the 1-monoglyceride of capric acid (monocaprin) with microbicidal activities against the food-borne bacteria Campylobacter jejuni, Salmonella spp., and Escherichia coli."

107. Assunção, "Effects of dietary coconut oil on the biochemical and anthropometric profiles of women presenting abdominal obesity."

108. Liau, "An open-label pilot study to assess the efficacy and safety of virgin coconut oil in reducing visceral adiposity."

109. Lieberman, "A review of monolaurin and lauric acid natural virucidal and bactericidal agents."

110. Biasi-Garbin, "Antifungal potential of plant species from Brazilian caatinga against dermatophytes."

111. Henderson, "Study of the ketogenic agent AC-1202 in mild to moderate Alzheimer's disease."

112. Ibid.

113. Newport, "A new way to produce hyperketonemia."

114. Francois, C. A., S. L. Connor, R. C. Wander, and W. E. Connor. 1998. "Acute effects of dietary fatty acids on the fatty acids of human milk." *American Journal of Clinical Nutrition* 67 (2): 301–8.

115. Liuba, P., J. Persson, J. Luoma, S. Ylä-Herttuala, and E. Pesonen. 2003. "Acute infections in children are accompanied by oxidative modification of LDL and decrease of HDL cholesterol, and are followed by thickening of carotid intima-media." *European Heart Journal* 24 (6): 515–21.

116. Huang, W. C., T. H. Tsai, L. T. Chuang, Y. Y. Li, C. C. Zouboulis, and P. J. Tsai. 2014. "Anti-bacterial and anti-inflammatory properties of capric acid against Propionibacterium acnes: a comparative study with lauric acid." *Journal of Dermatological Science* 73 (3): 232–40.

117. Srivastava, P., and S. Durgaprasad. 2008. "Burn wound healing property of *Cocos nucifera*: An appraisal." *Indian Journal of Pharmacology* 40 (4): 144–6.

118. Vysakh, "Polyphenolics isolated from virgin coconut oil inhibits adjuvant induced arthritis in rats through antioxidant and anti-inflammatory action."

119. Huang, "Anti-bacterial and anti-inflammatory properties of capric acid against Propionibacterium acnes."

120. Intahphuak, "Anti-inflammatory, analgesic, and antipyretic activities of virgin coconut oil."

121. Manuel-y-Keenoy, B., L. Nonneman, H. de Bosscher, J. Vertommen, S. Schrans, K. Klütsch, and I. De Leeuw. 2002. "Effects of intravenous supplementation with alpha-tocopherol in patients receiving total parenteral nutrition containing medium- and long-chain triglycerides." *European Journal of Clinical Nutrition* 56 (2): 121–8.

122. Conlon, L. E., R. D. King, N. E. Moran, and J. W. Erdman Jr. 2012. "Coconut oil enhances tomato carotenoid tissue accumulation compared to safflower oil in the Mongolian gerbil (Meriones unguiculatus)." *Journal of Agriculture and Food Chemistry* 60 (34): 8386–94.

123. Thormar, H., C. E. Isaacs, H. R. Brown, M. R. Barshatzky, and T. Pessolano. 1987. "Inactivation of enveloped viruses and killing of cells by fatty acids and monoglycerides." *Antimicrobial Agents and Chemotherapy* 31 (1): 27–31.

124. Hornung, B., E. Amtmann, and G. Sauer. 1994. "Lauric acid inhibits the maturation of vesicular stomatitis virus." *Journal of General Virology* 75 (Pt. 2): 353–61.

125. Ogbolu, "In vitro antimicrobial properties of coconut oil on Candida species in Ibadan, Nigeria."

126. Bergsson, G., J. Arnfinnsson, O. Steingrímsson, and H. Thormar. 2001. "In vitro killing of *Candida albicans* by fatty acids and monoglycerides." *Antimicrobial Agents and Chemotherapy* 45 (11): 3209–12.

127. Shinohara, H., H. Fukumitsu, A. Seto, and S. Furukawa. 2013. "Medium-chain fatty acid-containing dietary oil alleviates the depression-like behaviour in mice exposed to stress due to chronic forced swimming." *Journal of Functional Foods* 5 (2): 601–6.

128. Ogbolu, "In vitro antimicrobial properties of coconut oil on Candida species in Ibadan, Nigeria."

129. Bergsson, "In vitro killing of *Candida albicans* by fatty acids and monoglycerides."

130. Evangelista, M. T., F. Abad-Casintahan, and L. Lopez-Villafuerte. 2014. "The effect of topical virgin coconut oil on SCORAD index, transepidermal water loss, and skin capacitance in mild to moderate pediatric atopic dermatitis: a randomized, double-blind, clinical trial." *International Journal of Dermatology* 53 (1): 100–8.

131. Thormar, "Stable concentrated emulsions of the 1-monoglyceride of capric acid (monocaprin) with microbicidal activities against the food-borne bacteria Campylobacter jejuni, Salmonella spp., and Escherichia coli."

132. Aly, "Therapeutic effect of lauric acid, a medium chain saturated fatty acid, on Giardia lamblia in experimentally infected hamsters."

133. Römer, H., M. Guerra, J. M. Piña, M. Urrestarazu, D. García, and M. Blanco. 1991. "Realimentation of dehydrated children with acute diarrhea. com parison of cow's milk to a chicken-based formula." *Journal of Pediatric Gastroenterology Nutrition* 13 (1): 46–51.

134. Mutalib, Haliza Abdul, Sharanjeet Kaur, Ahmad Rohi Ghazali, Ng Chinn Hooi, and Nor Hasanah Safie. 2015. "A pilot study: the efficacy of virgin coconut oil as ocular rewetting agent on rabbit eyes." *Evidence-Based Complementary and Alternative Medicine* 2015: 135987.

135. Vysakh, "Polyphenolics isolated from virgin coconut oil inhibits adjuvant induced arthritis in rats through antioxidant and anti-inflammatory action."

136. Huang, "Anti-bacterial and anti-inflammatory properties of capric acid against Propionibacterium acnes."

137. Nakatsuji, Teruaki, Mandy C. Kao, Jia-You Fang, Christos C. Zouboulis, Liangfang Zhang, Richard L. Gallo, and Chun-Ming Huang. 2009. "Antimicrobial property of lauric acid against Propionibacterium acnes: its therapeutic potential for inflammatory acne vulgaris." *Journal of Investigative Dermatology* 129 (10): 2480–8.

138. Ibid.

139. Shinohara, "Medium-chain fatty acid-containing dietary oil alleviates the depression-like behaviour in mice exposed to stress due to chronic forced swimming."

140. Intahphuak, "Anti-inflammatory, analgesic, and antipyretic activities of virgin coconut oil."

141. Henderson, "Study of the ketogenic agent AC-1202 in mild to moderate Alzheimer's disease."

142. Newport, "A new way to produce hyperketonemia."

143. Shinohara, "Medium-chain fatty acid-containing dietary oil alleviates the depression-like behaviour in mice exposed to stress due to chronic forced swimming."

144. Duke, W. 2009. "Medicine: *Cocos nucifera* Folk Medicine."

145. DebMandal, "Coconut (Cocos nucifera L.: Arecaceae): In health promotion and disease prevention."

146. Arora, "Potential of complementary and alternative medicine in preventive management of novel H1N1 flu (swine flu) pandemic."

147. Projan, "Glycerol monolaurate inhibits the production of beta-lactamase, toxic shock toxin-1, and other staphylococcal exoproteins by interfering with signal transduction."

148. Abate, M. A., and T. L. Moore. 1985. "Monooctanoin use for gallstone dissolution." *Drug Intelligence and Clinical Pharmacy* 19 (10): 708–13.

149. Mumcuoglu, K. Y., J. Miller, C. Zamir, G. Zentner, V. Helbin, and A. Ingber. 2002. "The in vivo pediculicidal efficacy of a natural remedy." *The Israel Medical Association Journal* 4 (10): 790–3.

150. Burgess, I. F., E. R. Brunton, and N. A. Burgess. 2010. "Clinical trial showing superiority of a coconut and anise spray over permethrin 0.43% lotion for head louse infestation, ISRCTN96469780." *European Journal of Pediatrics* 169 (1): 55–62.

151. Huang, "Anti-bacterial and anti-inflammatory properties of capric acid against Propionibacterium acnes."

152. Assunção, "Effects of dietary coconut oil on the biochemical and anthropometric profiles of women presenting abdominal obesity."

153. Feranil, "Coconut oil is associated with a beneficial lipid profile in pre-menopausal women in the Philippines."

154. Ibid.

155. DebMandal, "Coconut (Cocos nucifera L.: Arecaceae): In health promotion and disease prevention."

156. Salam, R. A., G. L. Darmstadt, and Z. A. Bhutta. 2015. "Effect of emollient therapy on clinical outcomes in preterm neonates in Pakistan: a randomised controlled trial." *Archives of Disease in Childhood: Fetal Neonatal Edition* 100 (3): F210–15.

157. Marina, "Virgin coconut oil: emerging functional food oil."

158. Arunima, S., and T. Rajamohan. 2013. "Effect of virgin coconut oil enriched diet on the antioxidant status and paraoxonase 1 activity in ameliorating the oxidative stress in rats—a comparative study." *Food & Function* 4 (9): 1402–9.

159. Iranloye, "Anti-diabetic and antioxidant effects of virgin coconut oil in alloxan induced diabetic male Sprague Dawley rats."

160. Das, N. G., D. R. Nath, I. Baruah, P. K. Talukdar, and S. C. Das. 1999. "Field evaluation of herbal mosquito repellents." *Journal of Communicable Disease* 31 (4): 241–5.

161. Iranloye, "Anti-diabetic and antioxidant effects of virgin coconut oil in alloxan induced diabetic male Sprague Dawley rats."

162. Takahashi, M., S. Inoue, K. Hayama, K. Ninomiya, and S. Abe. 2012. "Inhibition of Candida mycelia growth by medium chain fatty acids, capric acid in vitro and its therapeutic efficacy in murine oral candidiasis." *Medical Mycology Journal* 53 (4): 255–61.

163. Bergsson, "In vitro killing of *Candida albicans* by fatty acids and monoglycerides."

164. Ogbolu, "In vitro antimicrobial properties of coconut oil on Candida species in Ibadan, Nigeria."

165. Sankaranarayanan, K., J. A. Mondkar, M. M. Chauhan, B. M. Mascarenhas, A. R. Mainkar, and R. Y. Salvi. 2005. "Oil massage in neonates: an open randomized controlled study of coconut versus mineral oil." *Indian Pediatrics* 42 (9): 877–84.

166. Francois, "Acute effects of dietary fatty acids on the fatty acids of human milk."

167. "Diet, Nutrition and Inflammatory Bowel Disease." 2013. Crohn's and Colitis Foundation of America: 5.

168. Manuel-y-Keenoy, "Effects of intravenous supplementation with alpha-tocopherol in patients receiving total parenteral nutrition containing medium- and long-chain triglycerides."

169. Conlon, "Coconut oil enhances tomato carotenoid tissue accumulation compared to safflower oil in the Mongolian gerbil (Meriones unguiculatus)."

170. Huang, "Anti-bacterial and anti-inflammatory properties of capric acid against Propionibacterium acnes."

171. Mutalib, "A pilot study: the efficacy of virgin coconut oil as ocular rewetting agent on rabbit eyes."

172. Zakaria, "Hepatoprotective activity of dried- and fermented-processed virgin coconut oil."

173. Otuechere, C. A., G. Madarikan, T. Simisola, O. Bankole, and A. Osho. 2014. "Virgin coconut oil protects against liver damage in albino rats challenged with the anti-folate combination, trimethoprim-sulfamethoxazole." *Journal of Basic Clinical Physiology and Pharmacology* 25 (2): 249–53.

174. Iranloye, "Anti-diabetic and antioxidant effects of virgin coconut oil in alloxan induced diabetic male Sprague Dawley rats."

175. Huang, "Anti-bacterial and anti-inflammatory properties of capric acid against Propionibacterium acnes."

176. Wruck, "Role of oxidative stress in rheumatoid arthritis."

177. Vysakh, "Polyphenolics isolated from virgin coconut oil inhibits adjuvant induced arthritis in rats through antioxidant and anti-inflammatory action."

178. DebMandal, "Coconut (Cocos nucifera L.: Arecaceae): In health promotion and disease prevention."

179. Bergsson, "In vitro killing of *Candida albicans* by fatty acids and monoglycerides."

180. Waldman, A., A. Gilhar, L. Duek, and I. Berdicevsky. 2001. "Incidence of Candida in psoriasis—a study on the fungal flora of psoriatic patients." *Mycoses* 44 (3–4): 77–81.

181. Ogbolu, "In vitro antimicrobial properties of coconut oil on Candida species in Ibadan, Nigeria."

182. Huang, "Anti-bacterial and anti-inflammatory properties of capric acid against Propionibacterium acnes."

183. Ibid.

184. Intahphuak, "Anti-inflammatory, analgesic, and antipyretic activities of virgin coconut oil."

185. Gracey, Michael, Valerie Burke, and Charlotte M. Anderson. 1970. "Medium Chain Triglycerides in Paediatric Practice." *Archives of Disease in Childhood* 45 (242): 445–52.

186. Lieberman, "A review of monolaurin and lauric acid natural virucidal and bactericidal agents."

187. Projan, "Glycerol monolaurate inhibits the production of beta-lactamase, toxic shock toxin-1, and other staphylococcal exoproteins by interfering with signal transduction."

188. Huang, "Anti-bacterial and anti-inflammatory properties of capric acid against Propionibacterium acnes."

189. Ogbolu, "In vitro antimicrobial properties of coconut oil on Candida species in Ibadan, Nigeria."

190. Takahashi, "Inhibition of Candida mycelia growth by medium chain fatty acids, capric acid in vitro and its therapeutic efficacy in murine oral candidiasis."

191. Bergsson, "In vitro killing of *Candida albicans* by fatty acids and monoglycerides."

192. Ogbolu, "In vitro antimicrobial properties of coconut oil on Candida species in Ibadan, Nigeria."

193. Schuster, G. S., T. R. Dirksen, A. E. Ciarlone, G. W. Burnett, M. T. Reynolds, and M. T. Lankford. 1980. "Anticaries and antiplaque potential of free-fatty acids in vitro and in vivo." *Pharmacology and Therapeutics in Dentistry* 5 (1–2): 25–33.

194. Peedikayil, F. C., V. Remy, S. John, T. P. Chandru, P. Sreenivasan, and G. A. Bijapur. 2016. "Comparison of antibacterial efficacy of coconut oil and chlorhexidine on Streptococcus mutans: an in vivo study." *Journal of International Society of Preventive and Community Dentistry* 6 (5): 447–52.

195. Fife, *Coconut Cures.*

196. Liau, "An open-label pilot study to assess the efficacy and safety of virgin coconut oil in reducing visceral adiposity."

197. Assunção, "Effects of dietary coconut oil on the biochemical and anthropometric profiles of women presenting abdominal obesity."

198. Lei, Tianguang, Weisheng Xie, Jianrong Han, Barbara E. Corkey, James A. Hamilton, and Wen Guo. 2004. "Medium-chain fatty acids attenuate agonist stimulated lipolysis, mimicking the effects of starvation." *Obesity Research and Clinical Practice* 12 (4): 599–611.

199. Kasai, "Comparison of diet-induced thermogenesis of foods containing medium- versus long-chain triacylglycerols."

200. Manuel-y-Keenoy, "Effects of intravenous supplementation with alpha-tocopherol in patients receiving total parenteral nutrition containing medium- and long-chain triglycerides."

201. Conlon, "Coconut oil enhances tomato carotenoid tissue accumulation compared to safflower oil in the Mongolian gerbil (Meriones unguiculatus)."

202. Nevin, K. G., and T. Rajamohan. 2010. "Effect of topical application of virgin coconut oil on skin components and antioxidant status during dermal wound healing in young rats." *Skin Pharmacology and Physiology* 23 (6): 290–7.

203. Huang, "Anti-bacterial and anti-inflammatory properties of capric acid against Propionibacterium acnes."

204. Agero, A. L., and V. M. Verallo-Rowell. 2004. "A randomized double-blind controlled trial comparing extra virgin coconut oil with mineral oil as a moisturizer for mild to moderate xerosis." *Dermatitis* 15 (3): 109–16.

205. Nakatsuji, "Antimicrobial property of lauric acid against Propionibacterium acnes."

206. Henry, "Antioxidant and cyclooxygenase activities of fatty acids found in food."

207. Marina, "Chemical properties of virgin coconut oil."

208. Nevin, "Effect of topical application of virgin coconut oil on skin components and antioxidant status during dermal wound healing in young rats."

209. Rele, A. S., and R. B. Mohile. 2003. "Effect of mineral oil, sunflower oil, and coconut oil on prevention of hair damage." *Journal of Cosmetic Science* 54 (2): 175–92.

210. Ruetsch, S. B., Y. K. Kamath, A. S. Rele, and R. B. Mohile. 2001. "Secondary ion mass spectrometric investigation of penetration of coconut and mineral oils into human hair fibers: relevance to hair damage." *Journal of Cosmetic Science* 52 (3): 169–84.

211. Ogbolu, "In vitro antimicrobial properties of coconut oil on Candida species in Ibadan, Nigeria."

212. Bergsson, "In vitro killing of *Candida albicans* by fatty acids and monoglycerides."

213. Ogbolu, "In vitro antimicrobial properties of coconut oil on Candida species in Ibadan, Nigeria."

214. Barnabé, W., T. de Mendonça Neto, F. C. Pimenta, L. F. Pegoraro, and J. M. Scolaro. 2004. "Efficacy of sodium hypochlorite and coconut soap used as disinfecting agents in the reduction of denture stomatitis, Streptococcus mutans and Candida albicans." *Journal of Oral Rehabilitation* 31 (5): 453–9.

215. Schuster, "Anticaries and antiplaque potential of free-fatty acids in vitro and in vivo."

216. Peedikayil, "Comparison of antibacterial efficacy of coconut oil and chlorhexidine on Streptococcus mutans."

217. Peedikayil, "Effect of coconut oil in plaque related gingivitis."

218. Mutalib, "A pilot study: the efficacy of virgin coconut oil as ocular rewetting agent on rabbit eyes."

219. Rele, "Effect of mineral oil, sunflower oil, and coconut oil on prevention of hair damage."

220. Ruetsch, "Secondary ion mass spectrometric investigation of penetration of coconut and mineral oils into human hair fibers."

221. Agero, "A randomized double-blind controlled trial comparing extra virgin coconut oil with mineral oil as a moisturizer for mild to moderate xerosis."

222. Nevin, "Effect of topical application of virgin coconut oil on skin components and antioxidant status during dermal wound healing in young rats."

223. Ogbolu, "In vitro antimicrobial properties of coconut oil on Candida species in Ibadan, Nigeria."

224. Bergsson, "In vitro killing of *Candida albicans* by fatty acids and monoglycerides."

225. Kaur, Chanchal Deep, and Swarnlata Saraf. 2010. "In vitro sun protection factor determination of herbal oils used in cosmetics." *Pharmacognosy Research* 2 (1): 22–5.

226. Ogbolu, "In vitro antimicrobial properties of coconut oil on Candida species in Ibadan, Nigeria."

227. Agero, "A randomized double-blind controlled trial comparing extra virgin coconut oil with mineral oil as a moisturizer for mild to moderate xerosis."

ABOUT THE AUTHOR

SUSAN BRANSON earned an undergraduate degree in biology from St. Francis Xavier University, then a MSc in toxicology from the University of Ottawa. From there, she worked in research: in the field, in the lab, as a writer, and as an administrator. She took time off and stayed at home after her second child was born. In addition to being a stay-at-home mom, she also took violin lessons, photography courses, earned a diploma in writing, and ultimately became a holistic nutritional consultant. Susan is a member of CSNN's Alumni Association, Canada's leading holistic nutrition school.

ABOUT FAMILIUS

VISIT OUR WEBSITE: WWW.FAMILIUS.COM
JOIN OUR FAMILY

There are lots of ways to connect with us! Subscribe to our newsletters at www.familius.com to receive uplifting daily inspiration, essays from our Pater Familius, a free ebook every month, and the first word on special discounts and Familius news.

GET BULK DISCOUNTS

If you feel a few friends and family might benefit from what you've read, let us know and we'll be happy to provide you with quantity discounts. Simply email us at orders@familius.com.

CONNECT

Facebook: www.facebook.com/paterfamilius
Twitter: @familiustalk, @paterfamilius1
Pinterest: www.pinterest.com/familius
Instagram: @familiustalk

FAMILIUS

THE MOST IMPORTANT WORK YOU
EVER DO WILL BE WITHIN THE
WALLS OF YOUR OWN HOME.

CPSIA information can be obtained
at www.ICGtesting.com
Printed in the USA
FSOW04n0414071017

9 781945 547157